"I am grateful to life

to my father

and to everyone who has helped me

...."

— Huang Ge

Say Thanks Before the End of Life

A True Story of a Great Father and a Strong Son

By Fang Wen

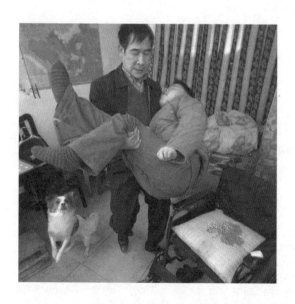

Foreign Languages Press

Project editor: Lan Peijin   Wen Fang

Text by: Fang Wen

Translated by: Sun Lei Yu Qiu

English text edited by: Solange Silverberg   Wang Guangqiang

First Edition 2008

Say Thanks Before the End of Life

—A True Story of a Great Father and a Strong Son

ISBN 978-7-119-05490-2

© Foreign Languages Press

Published by Foreign Languages Press

24 Baiwanzhuang Road, Beijing 100037, China

http://www.flp.com.cn

Distributed by China International Book Trading Corporation

35 Chegongzhuang Xilu, Beijing 100044, China

P.O. Box 399, Beijing, China

Printed in the People's Republic of China

Foreword

If you were someone with an incurable disease that would soon cut your life short, how would you spend your precious remaining days in this world?

If you were to have a sick child who needed full-time care and might leave you forever at any time, what would you do?

Whatever choice you were to make, people would likely be compassionate and understanding. Most people dying from a degenerative disease prefer to spend their last days peacefully. But a father with his sick son took the time to travel around China to say thanks to everyone who had helped them.

The father quit his job 12 years ago to take care of his son who has CMD (Congenital Muscular Dystrophy). As the boy's condition worsens, and their money drains, the man shores up hope and courage in their lives by fulfilling a wish of the son every year. The one he has just accomplished over the past three years is to bring the boy to every one of the many people in 80-plus cities in China who have helped them, in order to express their gratitude personally.

Only the power of the mind could provide the strength to enable a moribund boy and his distressed father to undertake such a journey, during which every day is a race against death. Living through the darkest and most bitter periods of life, the pair has repaid people for their kindness with brightness and hope. And here is their explanation.

Son: "Facing the end of my life, I find I have more wishes yet to be realized. My life is brief, so I treasure it more, and owe it greater gratitude…I receive help from others, but I never see them. This thought makes me feel ashamed, and prompts me to say "thank you" to them in person… A miracle is nothing but a work of man. It is unusual only because generally people think that adversity is too strong, and that they are too weak to overcome it."

Father: "A life doesn't have to be long, but it must be meaningful… I love my son very much, and am willing to make his life brilliant at any price… After experiencing so many things, we have come to a point where we are thankful for the care and support of many other people. Gratitude provides us with tremendous strength."

Feeling gratitude is the message the father and son disseminate during their cross-country tricycle trip. They strike the hearts of numerous people *en route* with the son's optimism and adamancy, the father's love and devotion, and the strength of human kindness. As a result more people are inspired to offer a helping hand to those in need, keeping the circle of giving and reciprocating endless.

As the son's life ticks to an end at a relentless unchanged pace, it grows more splendid, distinguishing its host from the average person.

Contents

I. Life's Countdown Started at the Age of 7

Huang Ge and his father Huang Xiaoyong live in a dilapidated bungalow in the Wangyuehu neighborhood, Rongwan Town, Changsha in Hunan Province.

The elder Huang, 48, ran a successful restaurant business before his son, 19, fell ill. He divorced when the boy was one, and from that time on assumed sole custody.

Huang Ge couldn't walk as steadily as other boys of his age when he was a toddler. The father however was not alarmed, presuming that this might be caused by slow growth. He began to worry about his son when the boy still experienced frequent falls at the age of three or four. But medical checks didn't uncover any problem with the boy's skeleton. The father then thought the cause might be a calcium deficiency, and so he intensified nutrition in the boy's diet. Despite such efforts, the boy's condition deteriorated steadily. After he groaned that he had "no strength in my legs" repeatedly when climbing steps, the father brought him to the hospital for a thorough examination. The results indicated that he had Congenital Muscular Dystrophy, a disease caused by a genetic defect for which a cure has not yet been found. The patients are expected to go through a painful progression of losing control of their muscles, a process which terminates when the heart stops and is followed by death, usually before the age of 18. Huang Ge was 7 that year.

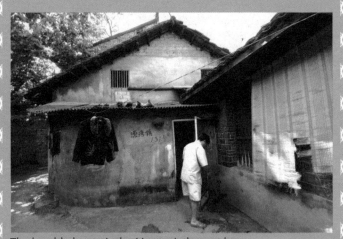

The humble house is the Huangs' pleasant home.

Full-time Dad

The news was a jolt from out of the blue for Huang Xiaoyong, knocking his mind blank for the moment. The man, known for his resilience and optimism to those close to him, didn't give up the hope that someday medical research would yield a cure for the disease, and spare his son from doom. Besides, he believed that his business could fund the boy's treat-

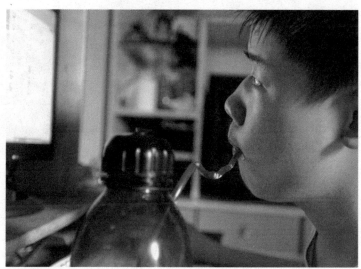

The father has tailor-made a bottle for his son with a straw that extends to the height of the boy's mouth.

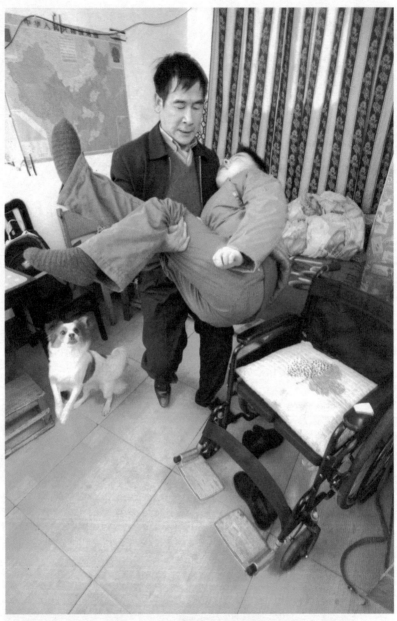

It is becoming increasingly difficult for the aging father to carry his son in and out of the wheelchair, but he never complains.

ment until a miracle occurred.

The father hid the truth from his son, and from that time on spent all of his time out of the office with him. Besides daily visits to the hospital, the father took the boy around the city and then throughout the nation to try every method that might help, including acupuncture, massage, *qigong* (*chi kung*) and even prayer in front of the Buddha. The costs accumulated to more than RMB 8,000 a month, but the boy's condition grew worse with each passing day.

The boy felt that he was getting weaker. Whenever he asked his father what was wrong with him, the answer was always malnutrition, and he was promised that he would be ok if only he ate more. While himself enduring heart-wrenching pain, the father put a smile on his face in front of his son, and worked out various lies to field the boy's questions.

In the third grade, Huang Ge's mobility reduced to the point that he could no longer move freely. He had to leave school for fear of imposing a burden on his classmates, who were often late for class after carrying him to the bathroom. On October 30, 1998, his tenth birthday, Huang Ge was no longer able to

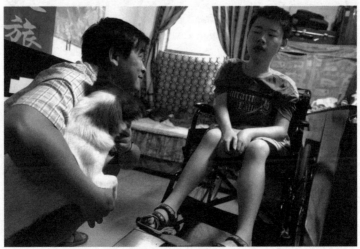

Papa used all means to make Huang Ge happy.

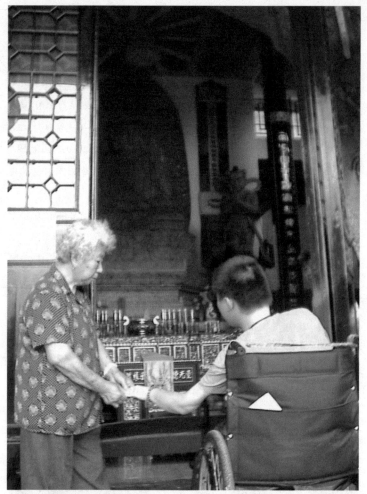

Huang Ge is taken to a temple in Yiwu, Zhejiang Province, to be treated for his illness.

walk, and received a wheelchair as a gift.

The son's deterioration didn't stop there. After turning pages and handling pens became increasingly difficult, the only thing he could do to kill time was to watch TV in his wheelchair, but the remote controller would slip out of his hand from time to time. At first he was taken care of by nannies. When he grew older and his temper grew shorter, it became difficult for a female outsider to accompany him, compelling his father to spend more time at home and inevitably less time on his business.

Finally, Huang Xiaoyong had to sell his restaurant.

With no income and the medical bills piling up, the elder Huang took a job driving a taxi. He worked only half-days, and left the boy to watch TV at home when he was out. One day he returned from work at noon, and was alarmed when he did not hear the usual greeting from his son. When he rushed to the living room, he saw the boy on the floor face down, his neck stuck in a chair, and at his last breath. When the father pulled him up, he tried to utter the word "dad," but couldn't make any sound. The father's tears poured down. He later learned that the boy had fallen from his seat while trying to retrieve the remote controller on the floor. This had happened before, but had never ended so dangerously. After this accident the father never dared to leave his son alone for long.

A man in the best years of his life gave up everything for the sake of his sick son. Nothing but a father's deep unselfish love could have prompted him to make such an enormous sacrifice.

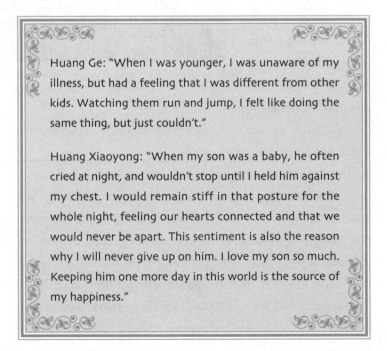

Huang Ge: "When I was younger, I was unaware of my illness, but had a feeling that I was different from other kids. Watching them run and jump, I felt like doing the same thing, but just couldn't."

Huang Xiaoyong: "When my son was a baby, he often cried at night, and wouldn't stop until I held him against my chest. I would remain stiff in that posture for the whole night, feeling our hearts connected and that we would never be apart. This sentiment is also the reason why I will never give up on him. I love my son so much. Keeping him one more day in this world is the source of my happiness."

Child of the Whole Neighborhood

Since selling their restaurant, the Huangs have been living in a rented home in Wangyuehu Residential Area. Though they are not registered permanent residents of the area, the neighborhood committee applied for

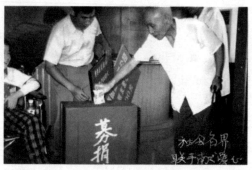

A donation is organized in Changsha for Huang Ge to cover his medical expenses, and draws the support of many corporations such as KFC.

the basic living allowance for them with the district government, which approved it as an exception.

The committee office is situated close to the Huangs' home. Committee members always call out Huang Ge's name when passing by, and check on his situation when hearing no response. One day Mrs. Sun found the boy flat on the ground. On another occasion Wang Peiru, Party Secretary of the committee, heard weeping in the room. He managed to open the door, and helped the boy back into his seat. "Don't let the motherless child feel ignored." This is the wish of every member of the community.

The Huangs' neighbors Mrs. and Mr. Yang shoulder the mission of providing the boy meals when his father is out. On bad weather days, their son and daughter-in-law take over the errand of bringing food to the boy, and watch him finish it. Another neighbor Mrs. Xia handles other chores, such as collecting clothes outdoors before it rains.

Whenever the elder Huang goes out, even for a couple of hours, he always leaves the key with his neighbors, asking them to keep an eye on his son. The neighbors can enter the Huangs' home whenever necessary.

Though the help from neighbors is often with the trivial things of daily life, it is heart-warming and evokes a sense of belonging and security for the father and son.

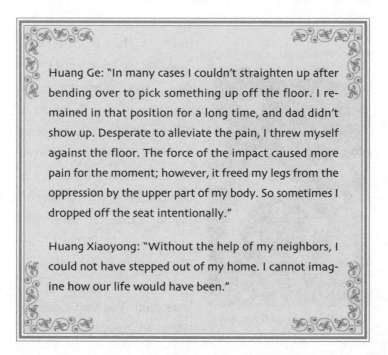

Huang Ge: "In many cases I couldn't straighten up after bending over to pick something up off the floor. I remained in that position for a long time, and dad didn't show up. Desperate to alleviate the pain, I threw myself against the floor. The force of the impact caused more pain for the moment; however, it freed my legs from the oppression by the upper part of my body. So sometimes I dropped off the seat intentionally."

Huang Xiaoyong: "Without the help of my neighbors, I could not have stepped out of my home. I cannot imagine how our life would have been."

Learning the Truth

One afternoon in 1999 Huang Xiaoyong left the boy, then 11, watching TV at home as usual while he was out. When he came back, the boy ranted at him: "Why didn't you tell me?" Pointing his finger to the TV set, he whined tearfully: "I watched the show True Feelings, and now know the cause of my illness." The stunned father realized the boy had learnt the truth, but had no idea how much he knew. That evening he watched the re-run of the program, which told the story of twin brothers in Xi'an with CMD. In covering the story the host expanded on the disease's symptoms and consequences. Wiping tears off the boy's face, the father tried to buoy him up: "Don't listen to this silly talk. With advances in science, every illness will have a cure. You have nothing to fear as long as I am with you."

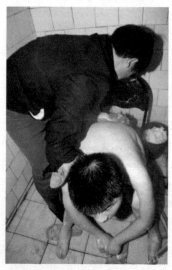

Giving the boy a bath is always an ordeal for the father.

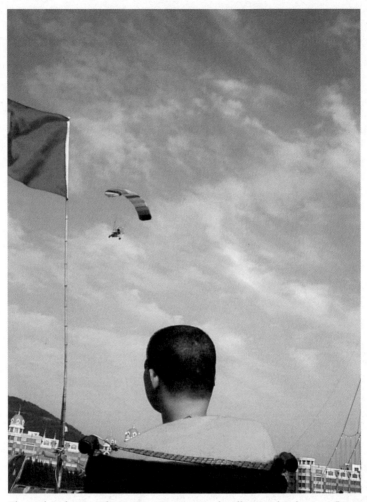

The sight of a parachute gives Huang Ge the illusion that he was flying with it.

The father believes that there is always hope for patients who keep their spirits up. Taking the words skeptically, the son calmed down.

For most children of 11, life has just unfurled its brilliance and promise. But Huang Ge's life was likely to end in seven years, a fact too cruel to be borne by any child of that age. He however saw no choice but to trust his father that a miracle might happen. The boy became an adult on that day.

The father felt unprecedented stress after his son discovered the gravity of his illness. As hiding him from reality had failed, the father worked to instill in his son a wise comprehension of disease and death. Whenever they encountered reports on car crashes and disasters, the father would comment: "See, a vibrant life may perish on any day. Life is as fickle as that. What we should cherish the most is what we have now. A life is not judged by its length but by its significance." The words inspired both the son and the father. The father began to think about what he could do to make his son's brief life more meaningful.

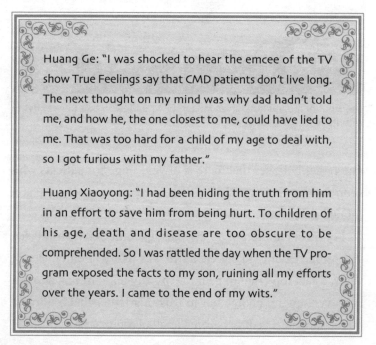

Huang Ge: "I was shocked to hear the emcee of the TV show True Feelings say that CMD patients don't live long. The next thought on my mind was why dad hadn't told me, and how he, the one closest to me, could have lied to me. That was too hard for a child of my age to deal with, so I got furious with my father."

Huang Xiaoyong: "I had been hiding the truth from him in an effort to save him from being hurt. To children of his age, death and disease are too obscure to be comprehended. So I was rattled the day when the TV program exposed the facts to my son, ruining all my efforts over the years. I came to the end of my wits."

A Flood of Love

    Knowing that his life was ticking to its end, Huang Ge missed his mother more than ever. On his 12th birthday he waited for his mother to show up, but was disappointed. He then asked for help from staff of the True Feelings show. On December 2, 2000, the Huangs were invited to the show, where they met the mother after years of absence. On the spot Huang Ge sang *Mother Is the Dearest in the World*, a ballad almost every Chinese child learns at an early age. The lady wept, so

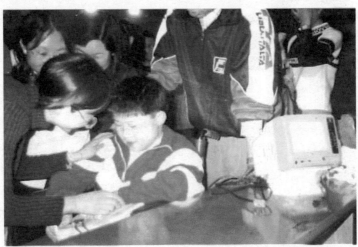

Young Huang Ge was very moved by the love of so many people.

did the audience in the room. But she refused to finally return to the family.

That night the program was aired to millions of homes throughout China. The Huangs' telephone didn't stop ringing from 10 pm to 2 am. People called to say kind words and offer help, but many were interrupted by sobs. In the following months, donations poured into the Huangs' home, with a total of 500 donations adding up to RMB 80,000.

A 19-year-old Miss Huang and three friends came to the Huangs' home at 11 pm the night the show was aired, sending the father and son all the RMB 2,300 in their purses, and urging the boy to fight his fate bravely. The second day the District Civil Affairs Office, Neighborhood Committee and some local enterprises brought a charity fund of RMB 20,000.

From December 3, 2000 on, people from around China and beyond flocked to the small home of the Huangs. For the first three or four days the number of visitors, many in families, exceeded 1,000. The Huangs had to ask their neighbors to help

Letters flooded in after the story of the Huangs was revealed by the media.

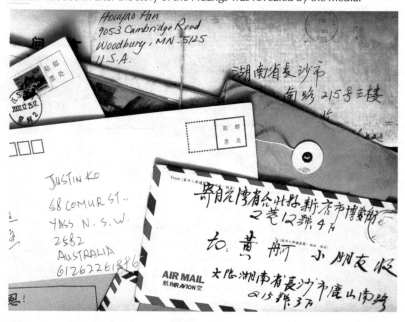

organize the long queues. People waited patiently, and came into the room group by group.

Learning on the show that Huang Ge had never been to KFC, a grandma in the city who was in her 70s arrived at the fast food chain at 6 am the next morning, without knowing that the store opened at 9. After three hours of waiting, she bought the meal and hot milk, and then shopped for a vacuum container for the drink, thinking it would be cold when it finally reached the boy. She boarded a bus, but mistakenly got off two stops earlier than she should have. It was noon when she finally found her way to the Huangs' home. On entering the house, she took the food out of the bag, saying: "My boy, here is the KFC. If you like it, I will buy you more next time." Everyone present was moved to tears by the scene.

Another 70-year-old lady, Mrs. Peng from the neighboring city of Zhuzhou, insisted on seeing Huang Ge personally after seeing the TV program, and refused to eat when her children, who worried about her health, tried to stop her from doing so. Her children finally rented a vehicle, and accompanied the lady to the Huang's home more than 100 kilometers away.

A Chinese American saw the program via CCTV's international channel. He immediately called his brother in China to send Huang Ge RMB 3,000 on his behalf. Chinese Australian Gao Zhiqiang sent his sister Gao Wenfang in Hong Kong to see Huang Ge, bringing him RMB 6,000 and many nutritional supplements and toys.

Meanwhile the father and son received loads of letters from around the nation and beyond. A Mrs. Li Wei in the U.S wrote: "We planned to eat out last weekend for my mother's birthday. That afternoon we watched your story on TV. My mother then refused to go out for the meal, so that the money could be saved to help Huang Ge. I tried to persuade her that I could afford both the party and the donation for the boy. But mom wouldn't give in. So I enclose a US $100 bill in this letter. Please accept the regards from a 70-year-old lady and her family."

Every piece of mail brought tears to the eyes of the father and son. They managed to write down more than 500 names and addresses they could obtain of these kind people.

Aiding people in need is traditionally deemed a virtue in Chinese culture. For those in dire situations, even a kind word can rekindle the flame in the heart, not to mention the visits by people coming from far away. The concerns and support the many strangers lavished on the Huangs strengthened their hearts, and lent them courage to surmount their challenges in life.

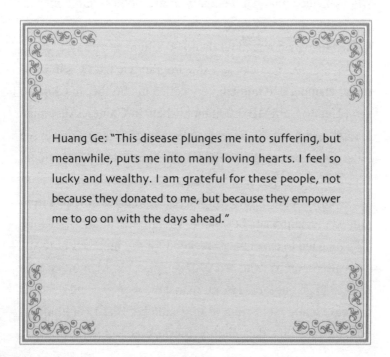

Huang Ge: "This disease plunges me into suffering, but meanwhile, puts me into many loving hearts. I feel so lucky and wealthy. I am grateful for these people, not because they donated to me, but because they empower me to go on with the days ahead."

Street Peddler

The public donations were a great relief for the father and son, but were utterly inadequate to sustain the costly medical treatment that the boy was undergoing. As the father had to look after the son day and night, taking a job became impossible. Their only income was the monthly RMB 260 basic living allowance from the government, with which they could not pay for both their house and for food.

The poster the Huangs display when they solicit help in the street.

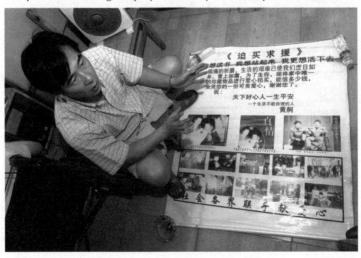

On May 1, 2002, the Labor Day holiday, as other families considered where to shop or seek out fun, the Huangs were confronted with the question of how to keep the pot boiling. "Dad, I am hungry. What do we have for breakfast?" The boy asked. The family had been living on porridge and fermented bean curd for a long period. Reaching deep into his pocket but finding not a single cent, the father agonized at the thought that they might starve that day. "Dad will take you out to find a way." He wrote about their situation on a large piece of paper and attached some photos. He then rolled the boy out of their home with some discs of the True Feelings show about their story and toys that people had sent to the boy, which he intended to sell on the street.

Hesitant and bashful, the father roamed the streets pushing the son's wheelchair, unable to find an appropriate place to start the business. He felt humiliated by his semi-selling semi-begging attempts. When they arrived at the Wuyi Square after roaming around for three hours without breakfast, the pair couldn't

Dilapidated home

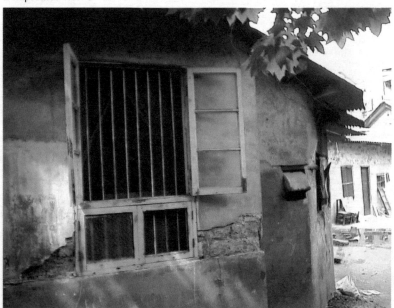

gather any further strength to walk on. At a quiet corner of the square, the father unfurled the paper, and displayed his commodities, silently waiting for buyers. Though there were few people around, everyone who passed by stopped to read the message, and then reached for their pockets. Some randomly took an item on offer, and some didn't take anything after leaving their money. In this way the father and son collected approximately RMB 90 that day, with which they managed for nearly 20 days with utmost thrift.

In the following six months such sales became the only means of living for the father and son. The pair, however, never went to the street until their last cent had run out, and insisted on selling instead of begging in a desperate effort to maintain their dignity. The sight of them was a reminder to people in the city of how strong man can be under the wheel of misfortune.

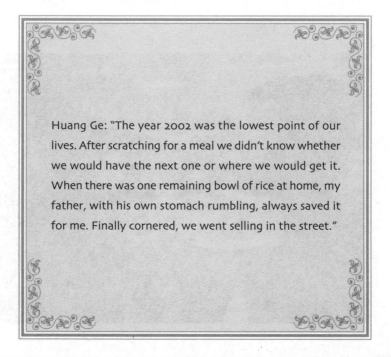

Huang Ge: "The year 2002 was the lowest point of our lives. After scratching for a meal we didn't know whether we would have the next one or where we would get it. When there was one remaining bowl of rice at home, my father, with his own stomach rumbling, always saved it for me. Finally cornered, we went selling in the street."

A Suicide Attempt

By the beginning of 2003, the family's financial situation had not improved in the slightest. Chronically sedentary, the son had grown into a flabby chunk of 55 kilograms, a weight too heavy for his father to carry. One night when carrying him to bed, the father broke his wrist. The accident was the last straw for the man ground down by eight years of such a harsh

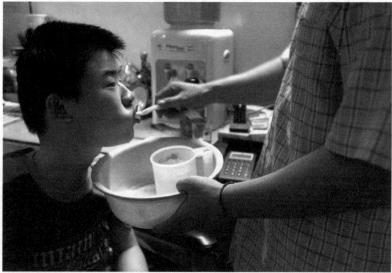

The father brushes his son's teeth.

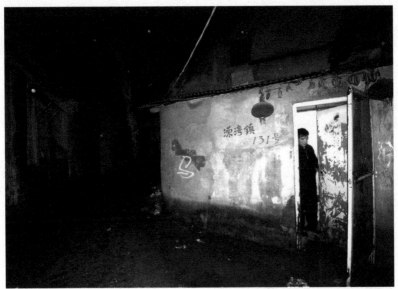

The father's spirits at a low point.

life. Seeing no light at the end of the tunnel and remembering the rent still to be paid for the second half of the year, the father burst into tears.

After the boy fell asleep, the father took a walk outdoors. He remembered a distant uncle in Zhuzhou City, and got the idea of borrowing some money from him. Huang Xiaoyong immediately headed for Zhuzhou with RMB 50 borrowed from friends, only to find the man had moved from his old address. Having no money and knowing nobody in the city, Huang wandered in the streets for the whole night. A drizzle further dampened his mood. Remembering his sick child and steep debts, he eventually lost the courage to go on with life. Exhausted and hungry, Huang climbed to the top of a seven-story building.

A crowd soon gathered below, and in no tome the police also arrived on the site. Among the anxious spectators were a few schoolchildren, the sight of whom reminded Huang of his son, which immediately cooled his head. "I am unfortunate, but my son is the most unfortunate one in the world."

The policemen pulled the rain-soaked Huang back from the

edge of the building. On learning his situation, they comforted him, and made a donation for his son when sending him off. Many people looking on in the crowd, which choked the road by the building, persuaded him to look on the bright side of things.

In his home in Changsha, during this time Huang Ge hadn't seen his father for a week, and had no idea where he had gone. The local TV station aired a notice looking for the missing father. And the neighborhood committee stepped in to help with house-keeping and cooking for the boy. When Huang Xiaoyong returned to see his home neat and his son sound, he felt ashamed of his cowardice, and reinforced his resolve to brave his life no matter how grim it might be.

A writer once said: On surviving despair people will find a new beautiful world. After the suicide incident, Huang Xiaoyong found greater passion for life, both his and his son's, and came closer to its meaning.

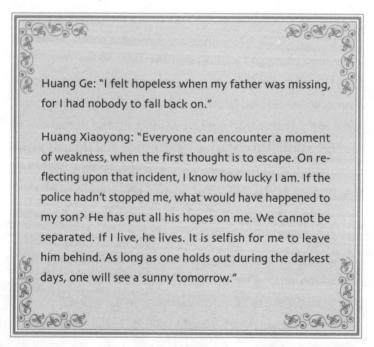

Huang Ge: "I felt hopeless when my father was missing, for I had nobody to fall back on."

Huang Xiaoyong: "Everyone can encounter a moment of weakness, when the first thought is to escape. On re-flecting upon that incident, I know how lucky I am. If the police hadn't stopped me, what would have happened to my son? He has put all his hopes on me. We cannot be separated. If I live, he lives. It is selfish for me to leave him behind. As long as one holds out during the darkest days, one will see a sunny tomorrow."

II. Pedal a Tricycle to Tian'anmen Square

Beginning with the day when Huang Ge learned about his disease, Huang Xiaoyong took on the dual mission of tending to his physical needs, and in the meanwhile, buoying up his spirits. He suggested that the boy make a wish every year, so that he would always have something to look forward to in life. Once there was a wish, the father would find a way to make it come true.

"I Want to See the Flag-Raising Ceremony in Tian'anmen Square"

In anticipation of realizing his dreams one by one, Huang Ge became sanguine, and often forgot the fact that he was wheelchair-bound. In the spring of 2001 he conceived the whimsical idea of attending the flag-raising ceremony in Tian'anmen Square in Beijing.

The idea baffled his father, who over the last several years had been watching palsy creeping all over the boy's body except for his neck and hands. Going on a trip of 2,000 kilometers seemed impossible for anyone in his situation. But on the other hand, he was tormented by the thought of having his son leave the world with unfulfilled desires. Huang Ge reasoned: "The future is unpredictable. Though the doctor has declared my fate, there is still a chance that it may go otherwise." Heartened by the boy's optimism, the father began to work to save money for their trip to Beijing.

The disease eroded Huang Ge's health more profoundly with the passing of every year. By the end of 2002, Huang Ge, feeling weaker than before, expressed once more his desire to go to Beijing at the earliest possible moment. Huang Xiaoyong knew that they couldn't wait any longer, and immediately began to plan for their transportation. Some people offered to fund their trip, but he declined, intent on making their trip an extraordinary one. "I am going to drive you to Beijing on a pedicab," he told the boy. "This method will be less comfortable, but will expose us to more marvelous scenes." Secretly he hoped he might find a remedy for his son's disease on the way. The boy didn't utter any objection to this plan. He didn't mind how they made their way to Beijing, as long as they could be there.

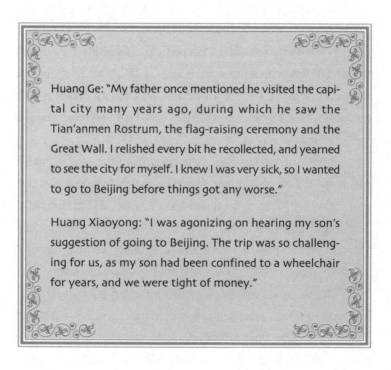

Huang Ge: "My father once mentioned he visited the capital city many years ago, during which he saw the Tian'anmen Rostrum, the flag-raising ceremony and the Great Wall. I relished every bit he recollected, and yearned to see the city for myself. I knew I was very sick, so I wanted to go to Beijing before things got any worse."

Huang Xiaoyong: "I was agonizing on hearing my son's suggestion of going to Beijing. The trip was so challenging for us, as my son had been confined to a wheelchair for years, and we were tight of money."

Setting out on a Rainy Day

After months of preparation, the father and son set their departure day for May 17, 2003, the Day of Help for the Disabled. Huang Xiaoyong retrofitted his pedicab, installing a cabin at the rear of the pedicab to seat Huang Ge in his wheelchair and to make room for objects of daily use, such as bedding and cooking wares. For a smoother ride, he added two more wheels to the vehicle.

Learning of the Huangs' departure from the media, many residents of Changsha came to see them off despite the heavy rain, bringing loads of food and travel outfits and giving their blessings. The small cabin was soon crammed full. Seeing Huang Ge cramped for space and imagining the long days he was to endure, an elder lady burst into tears on the spot.

With tears and rain drops streaming down his face, Huang Xiaoyong started up his pedicab, which was adorned with logos such as "My son, your father will accompany you through every test in life" and "I wish to live to 2008." He drove northward along the State Highway 107. Many people living *en route* followed their progress in the hopes of greeting the father and son in their native towns. Mrs. and Mr. Xu in Yueyang City

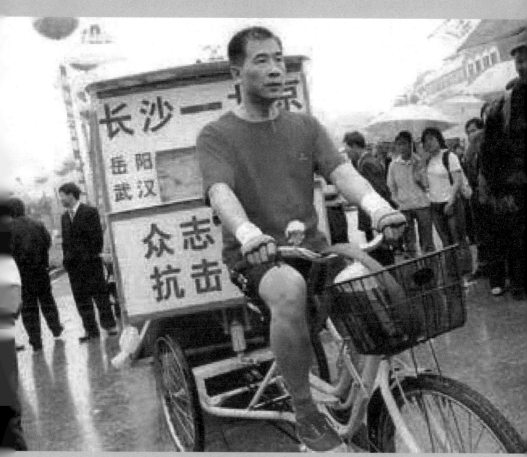

The father riding the tricycle-cart steadfastly through the rain waited for a dozen days by the highway before seeing the pair, and insisted on giving them a lavish treat at home.

When they left their home on May 17, 2003, Huang Xiaoyong and Huang Ge had little idea of the dramatic turn of events their Odyssey would bring to their lives. In the following three years they slogged on through one city after another on their beat-up pedicab.

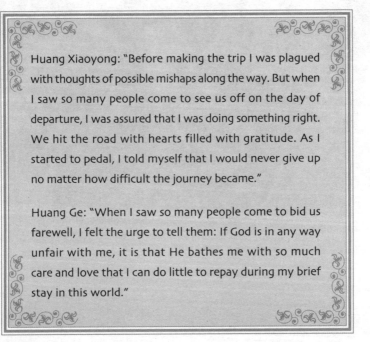

Huang Xiaoyong: "Before making the trip I was plagued with thoughts of possible mishaps along the way. But when I saw so many people come to see us off on the day of departure, I was assured that I was doing something right. We hit the road with hearts filled with gratitude. As I started to pedal, I told myself that I would never give up no matter how difficult the journey became."

Huang Ge: "When I saw so many people come to bid us farewell, I felt the urge to tell them: If God is in any way unfair with me, it is that He bathes me with so much care and love that I can do little to repay during my brief stay in this world."

A Day Is as Long as a Year

The pile of donated articles and the boy in the wheelchair added up to over 300 kilograms, a load too heavy for the father to manage. When his legs became extremely sore after lengthy periods of pedaling, the father shifted to hauling the vehicle with a thick jute rope, which left bruises on his shoulders and blisters all over his palms. He once broke two ropes in one day.

Rugged mountain roads could never thwart their advancing wheels.

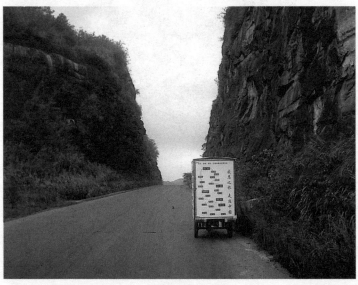

In the hot summer days there was little traffic on the curving highway that extended to the skyline. The journey seemed endless to the exhausted and dejected father, who strained every muscle towing the full overloaded carriage. In order to keep his spirits up, Huang Xiaoyong began to count the electricity poles lining the road at intervals of 50 meters. On passing every pole, he reminded himself that he was closer to success, and then had a short break before pushing on.

The father manages to fit his son and the wheelchair into their pedicab.

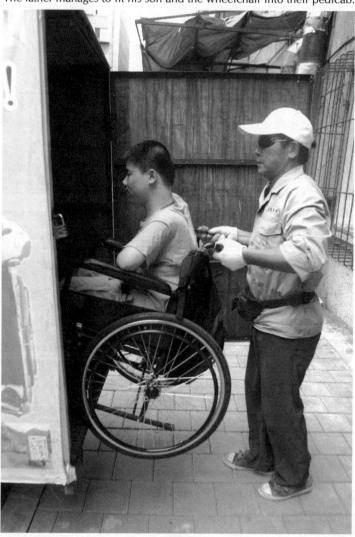

One day at dusk he was too exhausted to take another step. After pulling the pedicab over to the side of the road, he sat down against a rock, and immediately fell asleep. When he suddenly woke up at 9 pm, he jumped from the ground, and dashed over to check on his son. The boy, in summer shorts, had swelling mosquito bites dotted all over his exposed body. When the voracious bloodsuckers had attacked, Huang Ge couldn't lift a finger to drive them away, and furthermore, wouldn't disturb his sleeping father.

For much of the time the father and son were the only people on the road across rolling mountains. As the sun descended on the horizon, they often sat against a tree, admiring the splendid scene and exchanging encouraging words. On rainy days the father always stuck much of his own body out of the small cabin to leave more space for his son.

Many people have asked the following question: "Why did the Huangs go looking for so much trouble by making the long onerous trip? Wouldn't it have been nicer to stay in their cozy home?" For the son, no suffering would have been great enough to stop him from achieving his dream. For the father, nothing could stop him from honoring his words to help the boy reach his dream.

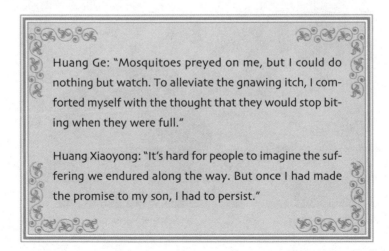

Huang Ge: "Mosquitoes preyed on me, but I could do nothing but watch. To alleviate the gnawing itch, I comforted myself with the thought that they would stop biting when they were full."

Huang Xiaoyong: "It's hard for people to imagine the suffering we endured along the way. But once I had made the promise to my son, I had to persist."

Getting Help Whenever They Were in Need

By the time that Huang Xiaoyong and Huang Ge arrived in the rural community Bishi in Yueyang, Hunan Province, the axle of their pedicab had broken under the heavy burden. The father had to bring the vehicle to a repair shop by the street. The photos and logos on the pedicab soon caught the attention of passers-by, who gathered around the father and son. Upon hearing their story, the crowd dispersed in silence. A woman

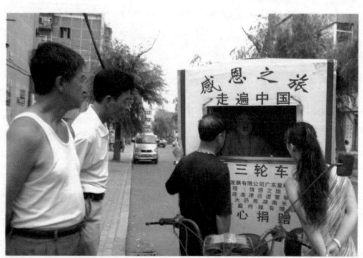

The Huangs' pedicab is eye-catching in the street throughout their Thanks-giving Journey.

later returned, tucking a wad of money into the father's hands, a donation the crowd had just made. The bills, new and old, and of various par values, moved the father and son to tears. These warm-hearted farmers were eager to do more for the pair. They bought a motorcycle, and moved the cabin from the pedicab to it. The engine power saved the father from the laborious pedaling, making his future days on the way much easier.

On a late May day the father and son arrived in a small town in Xianning, Hubei Province. When Huang Xiaoyong heaved his son in the wheelchair out of the cabin for lunch, the right wheel came off the chair, the result of a broken shaft. The wheel-

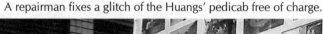
A repairman fixes a glitch of the Huangs' pedicab free of charge.

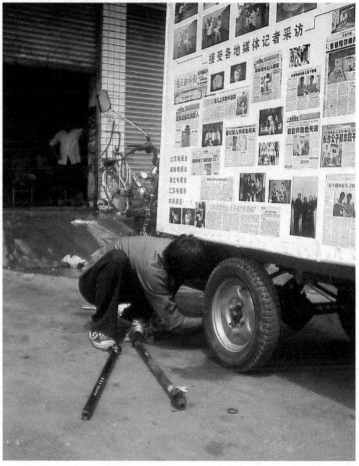

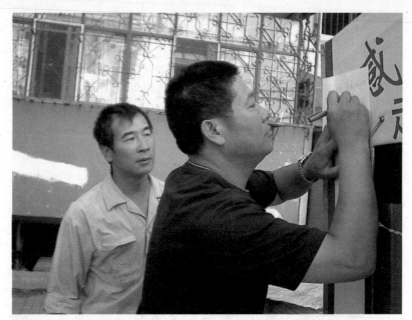

Meeting warm-hearted people along the way who took the initiative to keep in contact

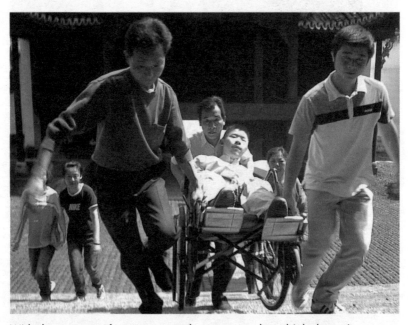

With the support of so many people, no matter how high the stairs, Huang Ge could climb them.

chair lurched, and got stuck at the gate of the cabin. After repeated futile efforts to pull it out, the father could hardly hold the wheelchair and his son on it any longer. At this moment a passer-by noticed this emergency, and yelled to other passers-by. Soon a dozen people came to assist. In minutes they had moved Huang Ge to a stool nearby, and brought him water. Two urban management patrols passing the site called in two other colleagues, and took the broken wheelchair to a repair shop.

The Huangs experienced countless mishaps with their motorcycle and wheelchair during their long and bumpy drive. But on every occasion they received help from local people wherever they went. The repairmen never charged a cent for their services, and spontaneously replaced any worn-out parts. Such acts of kindness always recharged the dog-tired father and son with fresh strength and courage.

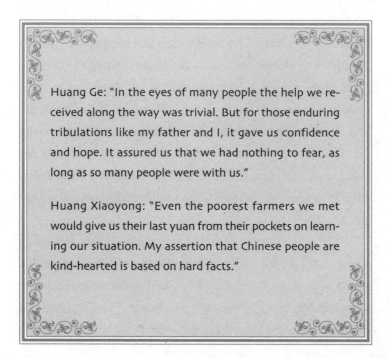

Huang Ge: "In the eyes of many people the help we received along the way was trivial. But for those enduring tribulations like my father and I, it gave us confidence and hope. It assured us that we had nothing to fear, as long as so many people were with us."

Huang Xiaoyong: "Even the poorest farmers we met would give us their last yuan from their pockets on learning our situation. My assertion that Chinese people are kind-hearted is based on hard facts."

Free Boarding in a Star Hotel

"When we arrive in Beijing, we should have a hearty meal of hometown dishes, and find a nice hotel." Huang Xiaoyong made this promise to his son along the way. Long periods of driving, erratic living and poor nutrition had depleted the pair's strength.

The day they eventually entered the suburbs of Beijing, they thought it was time for a celebration and some relaxation. A restaurant of Hunan cuisine by the street emitted the inviting smell of spicy food, which was hard to resist for the malnourished and home-sick father and son. There was a nice hotel, the Star Holiday Inn nearby, which still had a vacant room on the first floor. Despite the rate of RMB 288, Huang Xiaoyong decided to give his son the experience of a night in a star hotel. After checking-in, the pair went to the nearby restaurant for lunch.

When they returned to their room, the hotel manager and a dozen staff members were waiting for them at the door with a bunch of flowers. The manager insisted on refunding them the room deposit, saying: "We have just learnt your story. You can stay here as long as you like, and everything will be free." At an offer made out of genuine goodness, any attempt to refuse may have seemed ungracious. The Huangs stayed in the hotel for the following 36 days. During this period they visited various big hospitals in Beijing in search of a cure for Huang Ge's disease. After the news about the brave father and son had spread throughout the community, local residents flocked to their hotel to see them, and many took them to major tourist resorts in the city.

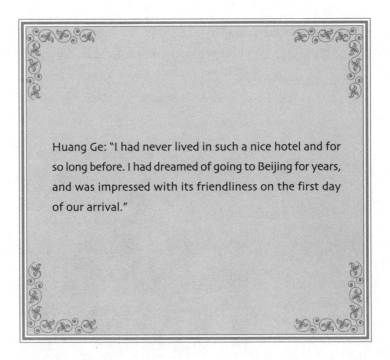

Huang Ge: "I had never lived in such a nice hotel and for so long before. I had dreamed of going to Beijing for years, and was impressed with its friendliness on the first day of our arrival."

Three Days of Extravagance

"Some businesspeople provided us help for reasons of publicity and their public image. But many others hid themselves from the media," commented the Huangs.

A successful businessman named Mr. Bai, who had a son of Huang Ge's age, felt obliged to help the unfortunate boy after reading the media reports, and immediately sent his chief of staff Mr. Li to the hotel where the Huangs were staying. Mr. Li

A little boy also tries to offer a helping hand when he meets Huang Ge in the street.

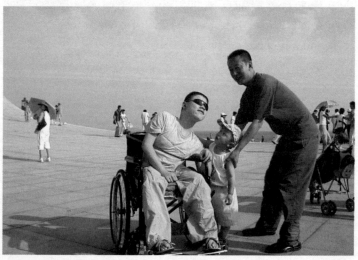

arrived when the father and son were at an interview with several members of the media. He didn't approach them until hours later after all the journalists had left. "My boss has sent me here, and told me not to get the media involved. We understand it is not easy to make the trip to Beijing in your manner, and we hope we can make your stay here more enjoyable. In the following three days we are going to give you a car with a driver, and we will satisfy all of your demands, such as what you feel like eating or which scenic spot you want to visit."

An 8-meter-long black limousine came to the hotel gate the

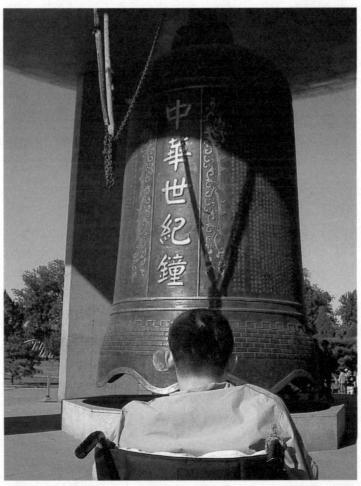

Huang Ge visiting the China Millennium Monument, fulfilling a long-held wish next morning, and the father and son started their three days of experience living like royalty. When the car pulled over at a posh restaurant for lunch at noon, all the guards and pageboys at the entrance came to greet what they expected to be a mogul, and were transfixed upon seeing a tanned boy and his tattered father in the back seat. The confusion and astonishment on their faces amused the Huangs. Regaining their composure, the staff helped the boy out of the car, and respectfully escorted the two into the restaurant.

The experience felt too good to be true for the father and son, who had been overwhelmed by destitution and illness for so long. They had never previously imagined that they might someday sample so many dainty dishes in one day and have entertainment normally available only to the very rich. The three days soon came to an end, but the flame of passion to strive for a happy life remained high in the Huangs' hearts. Throughout their untiring struggles with ill fate they relish every bit of joy and fun, and always look for the silver lining of every dark cloud.

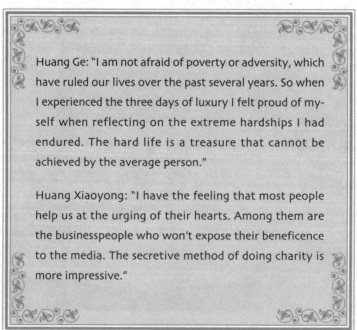

Huang Ge: "I am not afraid of poverty or adversity, which have ruled our lives over the past several years. So when I experienced the three days of luxury I felt proud of myself when reflecting on the extreme hardships I had endured. The hard life is a treasure that cannot be achieved by the average person."

Huang Xiaoyong: "I have the feeling that most people help us at the urging of their hearts. Among them are the businesspeople who won't expose their beneficence to the media. The secretive method of doing charity is more impressive."

Driving a Motorcycle to Tian'anmen Square

On the evening of July 20, the Huangs received a call from the Tian'anmen branch of the Beijing Municipal Public Security Bureau, which invited them to watch the flag-raising ceremony at Tian'anmen Square the next morning. They were told that the bureau had granted them a special permit to drive their motorcycle to the square on Chang'an Avenue.

The father and son set off early the next day. When they reached Chang'an Avenue, two police cars and a score of officers were waiting for them. The police escorted them all the way to the parking lot south of Tian'anmen. More officers in the region came to help Huang Ge out of the vehicle, and rolled him in his wheelchair to the best possible position to view the flag-raising ceremony. Under the rosy twilight the national anthem resonated, and as the awe-struck crowds gazed at the scene, the red five-star flag ascended slowly up the pole.

Huang Ge's eyes followed the movement of the flag, clasping a mini one in his feeble hand, unable to say anything more than "I am so happy." He had been waiting for this moment for

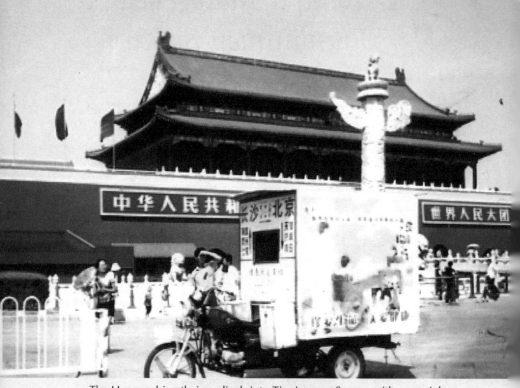

The Huangs drive their pedicab into Tian'anmen Square with a special permission.

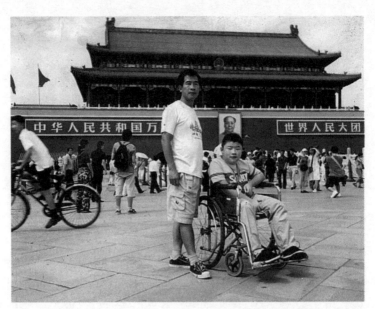

No matter what, Tian'anmen Square remains forever the home of their hearts.

so long. Tears burst from his eyes and from those of his father. Patriotism is a strong uniting force and also purifies the soul. It can only reside in a heart susceptible to kindness, unselfishness and other human virtues.

Huang Ge: "As the honor guard hoisted the red flag into the sky, all the people in the square stopped to watch in silence and respect. Inexpressible excitement and pride filled my heart. I believe this feeling was shared by everyone present."

Huang Xiaoyong: "The national anthem in the air and the flag above set my heart afire, igniting in me the passion to give my life for my motherland whenever necessary. At that moment I understood why my son had insisted on seeing the ceremony before the end of his life."

III. Giving Thanks Personally

The Huangs' journey to Tian'anmen Square was widely covered by the media. However, Huang Ge was perturbed by the use of grisly words such as "death" and "incurable disease" in the media reports. Growing weaker and weaker, the boy was aware that his time in this world was drawing to an end.

Sometimes he asked himself what death would be like, and shuddered at the thought that he would never see his family or anybody who cared about him again. While he was in Beijing, Huang Ge continued to feel that he owed something to the many people who had helped him. So he asked his father: "Dad, could we make use of the remaining time in my life to meet the people who aided us, and thank them in person?" It was a request the father could not refuse.

They opened the notebook in which they had been keeping records of donations they had received and made plans for their Thanksgiving Journey. They decided to complete it on three trips.

The First Thanksgiving Journey

In August 2003, the father and the son started their first Thanksgiving Journey from Beijing, bringing with them the notebook that recorded the name and address of their donors.

Time: August 26, 2003 to September 18, 2003

Length: 3700 kilometers

Route: Beijing-Tianjin-Cangzhou-Dezhou-Jinan-Zibo-Weifang-Qingdao-Rizhao-Lianyungang-Yancheng-Nantong-Shanghai-Hangzhou-Shangrao-Nanchang-Zhuzhou-Changsha

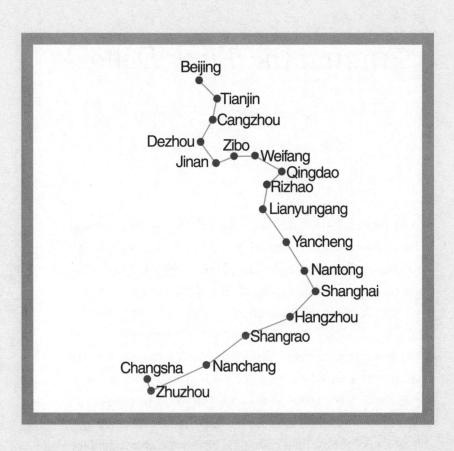

Finding the First Donor

In August 2003, the Huangs set their feet on the ground of Tianjin, where, a lady named Guan Qi, who had sent them a remittance of RMB 300 years ago, lived. Perplexed by the roads and lanes densely intersecting in the city they had never before visited, the father and son thought it would be better to seek the help of the locals. The father called the hotline of the most widely-read newspaper in Tianjin *Tonight* (*Jinwanbao*). A young journalist answered the phone, and was glad to be the Huangs' guide in their search for Mrs. Guan. The young man, however, was a recent graduate who had moved to the city not long ago. It took until the evening before the three were able to find the address specified on the remittance document. But to their disappointment, the lady had moved away. The news was a blow to them as they had been eagerly anticipating the meeting, but they would not give up hope. Huang Xiaoyong and the journalist knocked on the doors on every floor of the apartment building, asking the neighbors if anyone had Mrs. Guan's new address. But the answer was always no.

When they returned to Huang Ge, who was waiting outside of the building, it was very dark outside. Residents in the com-

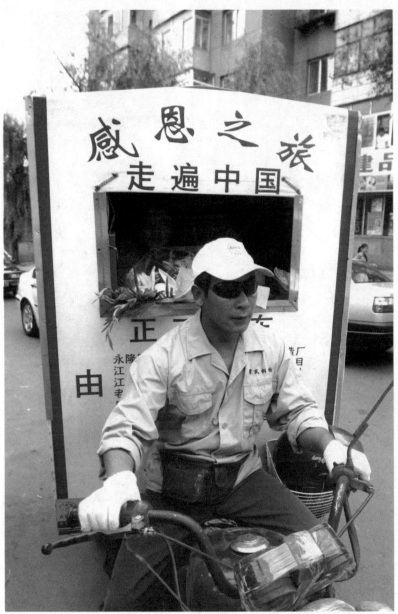

感 恩 之 旅
走遍中国

正

永隆

由

江江老

Fully outfitted, his father looking like a professional driver

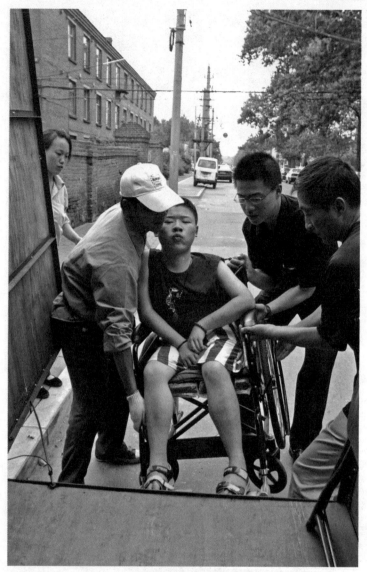
Helping hands assisting his father to lift Huang Ge onto the tricycle-cart

munity gradually gathered around the father and his handicapped son. After the father and son told their story, many residents said they knew Guan Qi, who was always ready to help
others. Suddenly an old peddler in the crowd said: "Are you
looking for Guan Qi? I have her number." At the Huangs'
request, he called Mrs. Guan, telling her that "a father and his

son whom you helped are now at you former residence to see you." On hearing this news, the first thought in Guan's mind was "that's impossible." But she immediately rushed to the site in a taxi.

The Huangs had never seen Mrs. Guan, but spotted her from afar when they saw a woman coming in their direction, sobbing. Guan never expected the father and son in Hunan Province who had received RMB 300 from her to travel more than a thousand miles to her home just to thank her. She held Huang Ge's hands, amazed to see that the boy was more cheerful and mature than he had been three years before, when he appeared in the TV show True Feelings. Huang Ge presented Guan with a bouquet of flowers, and took a picture with her.

In the following days of their Thanksgiving Journey the Huangs expressed their gratitude to every donor in this way. A bouquet of flowers is no expensive gift, but conveys deep feelings, as it is from a father and his son who have come from thousands of miles on a motorcycle.

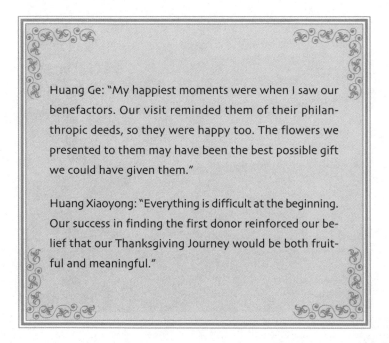

Huang Ge: "My happiest moments were when I saw our benefactors. Our visit reminded them of their philanthropic deeds, so they were happy too. The flowers we presented to them may have been the best possible gift we could have given them."

Huang Xiaoyong: "Everything is difficult at the beginning. Our success in finding the first donor reinforced our belief that our Thanksgiving Journey would be both fruitful and meaningful."

Seeing the Sea for the First Time

It was around 5 pm when the Huangs arrived in the coastal city Qingdao in Shandong Province. Having yearned to see the sea for a long time, they rushed to the shore without stopping to rest.

When the cerulean ocean eventually appeared in front of

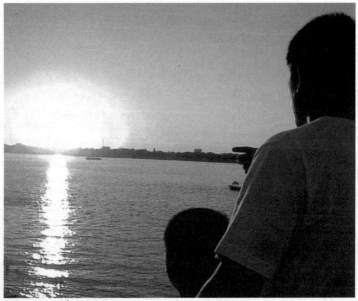

Sunset over the ocean.

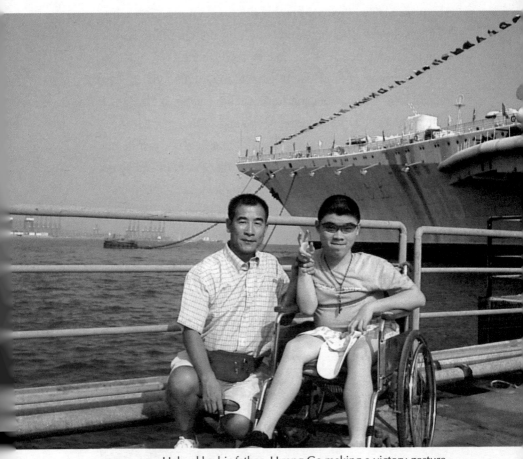

Helped by his father, Huang Ge making a victory gesture.

them, Huang Ge was elated, and was amazed to see the pier that extends over the waves. "Is it really erected out of the water?" He asked. The father was just as excited. He brought some seawater in his hands, and splashed it over the boy. Huang Ge tasted the drops on his lips, exclaiming, "It's salty." Feeling the moist breeze and watching the chopping waves, Huang Ge beamed with a sense of fulfillment.

On learning of the Huangs' arrival in Qingdao, the general manager of the local oceanarium, Zhao Fasheng, invited them to tour the park as VIP guests. At the end of the tour, Mr. Zhao sent the boy a dolphin toy and RMB 500 as a gift. Clasping the cute dolphin, Huang Ge expressed his thanks again and again.

Seeing the father leaping in the sea like a child and the son wearing smiles as bright as sunshine, people could hardly believe the pair had been through so many sorrows and distressful times. No matter how gloomy life might look, they always managed to keep their eyes open for any small thing that could bring them joy everyday. Facing the rolling ocean, they let the waves rush all the unhappy thoughts out of their minds.

He loves the sea because it is so expansive and tolerant.

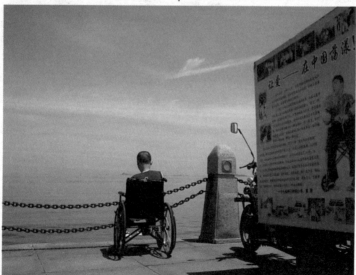

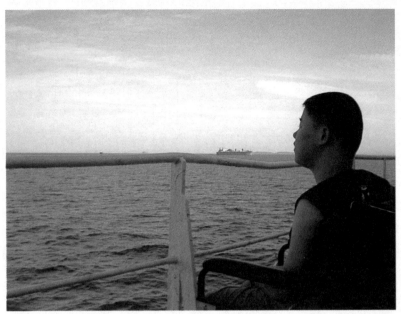
Gazing out at his dreams on the horizon.

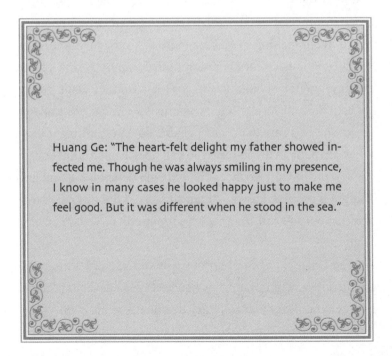
Huang Ge: "The heart-felt delight my father showed infected me. Though he was always smiling in my presence, I know in many cases he looked happy just to make me feel good. But it was different when he stood in the sea."

Encountering Suspicion

The Huangs began their search for their donors on their second day in Qingdao. When they came to the address of one of the donors, the two elders in the doorway, with heightened watchfulness, denied they knew the person. Huang Xiaoyong understood how people would be alarmed in the first instance when two ragged strangers showed up at their door.

To avoid making the elders more anxious, the father and son waited outside for the return of their donor. It was late in the day, and they couldn't wait for long. So they again asked for help from the local media. A reporter soon came, and showed his journalist's card to the elders in the doorway, asking if they knew anybody in the family who had once helped a father and his son in Hunan Province. The old lady called her daughter, and got a positive answer. "I am so sorry, I didn't know anything about her aid for you." She immediately showed the Huangs in.

The Huangs were not upset by this incident. It is normal that people who give out a few hundreds yuan never expect the recipient far away to thank them personally years later. When this does happen, the first response of many donors might be

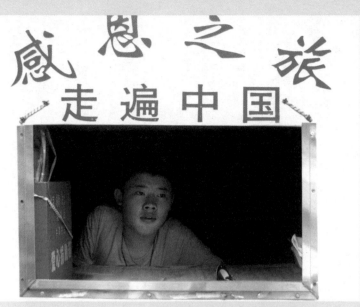

Huang Ge's eyes filled with hope for the future.

the question, "Is he/she seeking more money from me?" When they dispelled such skepticism with their deeds, the Huangs believed they could prove the extraordinary nature of their Thanksgiving Journey.

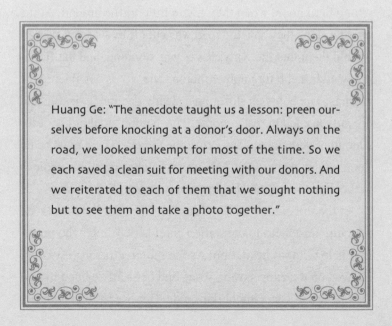

Huang Ge: "The anecdote taught us a lesson: preen ourselves before knocking at a donor's door. Always on the road, we looked unkempt for most of the time. So we each saved a clean suit for meeting with our donors. And we reiterated to each of them that we sought nothing but to see them and take a photo together."

A Flood Emergency

On September 8, 2003, the Huangs arrived in Lianyungang in Jiangsu Province. Eager to go home as soon as they could, they got up early in the morning, and hit the road immediately after breakfast. In their haste they ignored a notice board at the entrance of State Highway 204, saying "Flooding has severed the road, take a detour." They didn't realize something was wrong until noon, when they found little traffic around. At the top of a slope they saw the road was cut off by water. A passer-by told them that the Xinyi River was flooding, and the flooding wouldn't ebb for another month. The words bewildered the Huangs. The boy was suffering a steady decline in health, and urgently needed to rest at home. They simply couldn't wait for a month. Suddenly an idea struck the father: "There must be no flood on the expressway." He immediately steered his pedicab in the direction of the Nanjing-Lianyungang Expressway.

At the toll station of the Guanyun Exit, the father relayed their circumstances to the station chief Mrs. Wang, who promised help without hesitation. As the motored pedicab was not allowed on the expressway, Wang and her staff decided to find the father and son a hitchhiking ride. But over a four-hour period they weren't able to find a vehicle on the road with enough space for the bulky pedicab. As a last resort, Mrs. Wang called the local police patrol for help. The patrol team soon sent officers with a police car. It was now dark, so the police car turned on its lights, and escorted the slow pedicab down the expressway. It took them a full hour to complete the 37 kilometers. When they departed, the officers emptied their pockets to raise RMB 40, and asked the boy to buy some food with the money.

The photo of these officers is still on the wall of the Huangs' home. The father and son feel indebted whenever they see it, as they don't know the names of any of the officers. They asked, but the officers wouldn't tell them. But the two beams of their car lights left marks on the Huangs' memories, and would penetrate through every dark moment in their life.

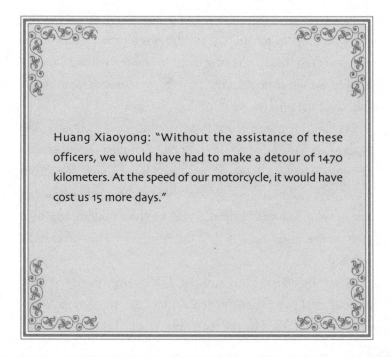

Huang Xiaoyong: "Without the assistance of these officers, we would have had to make a detour of 1470 kilometers. At the speed of our motorcycle, it would have cost us 15 more days."

A Special Mid-Autumn Festival

During the Mid-Autumn Festival of 2003, the Huangs entered Shanghai exurb, and considered having a sightseeing tour around the metropolis after meeting their donors there. They drove down State Highway 320, and soon headed into a busy district. A traffic officer stopped them at a crossroad, telling them that motored pedicabs were not allowed in the downtown area. The Huangs turned around, and saw police officers on the way back too. Understanding the rule and not willing to make trouble for the officers, they decided to stop and wait on the spot until the officers went off duty at 9 pm.

As the full moon crept to the zenith of the canopy, the Huangs, exhausted and hungry, imagined the jubilant scenes of family reuniting in other homes, and missed their own, from which they had been away for more than three months. Whether east or west, home is the best. At the moment nothing appealed more to the father and son than the thought of a hot meal and a soft bed.

After the officers left at 9 pm, the Huangs mounted their pedicab, and proceeded hurriedly out of the urban area. When rural scenes flashed by the road, they stopped at a small eatery to fill their growling stomachs. The food was awful, but was supposed to be a festival feast. It was past 11 pm when they got back to their vehicle, and they weren't able to find lodgings until 1 am.

The Huangs' homesickness grew ever stronger after this special Mid-Autumn Festival, a day that Chinese people traditionally spend with their families. The father and son decided to suspend their Thanksgiving Journey for some time, and have a break at home.

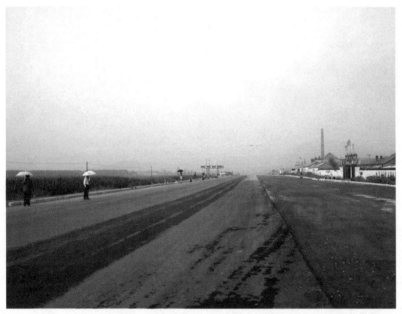

Enduring the hardship and exhaustion of a long journey.

The nearer they came to their home the more enthusiastic they became. After having quickly covered over 300 kilometers in 14 hours from 6 am to 8 pm on September 18, they were eventually back in downtown Changsha. When the father pulled over and looked around to his son, both burst out laughing: they looked as squalid as two miners just back to the surface. The father took a bottle of water, and they washed the dust off their faces before driving toward their home.

Home is always where a traveler's thoughts drift along the way. This was particularly true with the Huangs. Nothing looked more beautiful to them than their nest in their shabby house, where they had gone through all the good and bad experiences of life together. On reaching their front door, the father and son concluded their first Thanksgiving Journey.

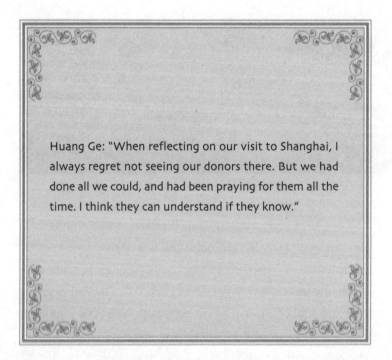

Huang Ge: "When reflecting on our visit to Shanghai, I always regret not seeing our donors there. But we had done all we could, and had been praying for them all the time. I think they can understand if they know."

The Second Thanksgiving Journey

In the early autumn of 2005, the Huangs resumed their Thanksgiving Journey. Before their departure they solicited 20 talismans at the Kaifu Temple in Changsha, which they intended to give their donors. Hong Kong was planned as one leg on their trip. When the father started up their vehicle, Huang Ge yelled: "Let's go! The destination – Hong Kong." (They ultimately didn't make it to the special administrative region as they had not completed the entry procedures.)

Time: September 10 to November 27, 2005

Length: 2700 kilometers

Route: Changsha-Hengyang-Chenzhou-Yizhang-Pingshi-Shaoguan-Guangzhou-Dongguan-Shenzhen-Zhuhai, then back to Changsha by the same route

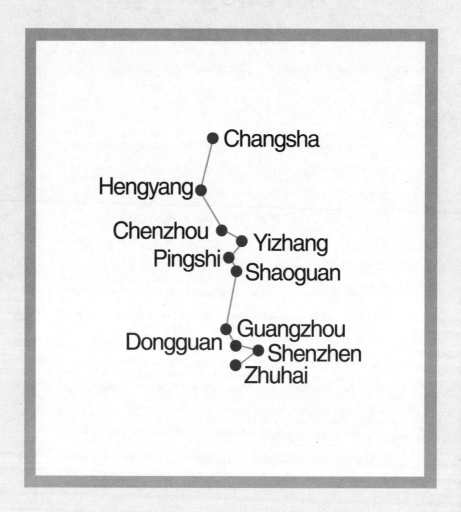

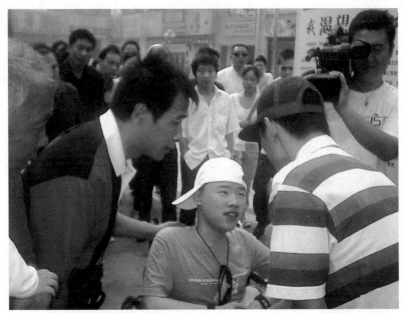

Crowds of Changsha residents see the Huangs off on their second Thanksgiving Journey.

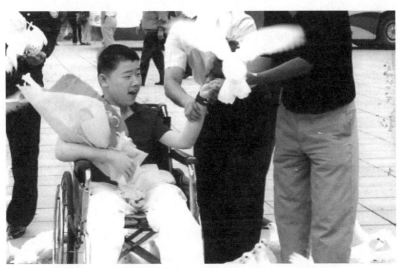

Warm-hearted people helping Huang Ge hold pigeons.

Losing the Pedicab

The Huangs never thought of the possibility of someday having their beat-up pedicab stolen. But it did disappear overnight during their stay in Dongguan, Guangdong Province, together with all the records of their previous trips around China. These records would have been of little value to other people, but were priceless to the Huangs.

The father had seldom locked the vehicle during their trips, as the idea of "stealing" had never crossed his mind. "When it did happen, I couldn't find an explanation," said the elder Huang. But he had to hide his bitterness, and tried to reduce to a minimum the blow from this incident for the sake of his son.

As the pair was worrying about how to complete the rest of their journey, a local resident named Mr. Han Rengen, who had helped the Huangs years earlier, learnt of the incident through the media, and immediately came to help. He sent them RMB 3,000, and what's more, drove them around the city and to the neighboring cities of Guangzhou and Zhuhai over the

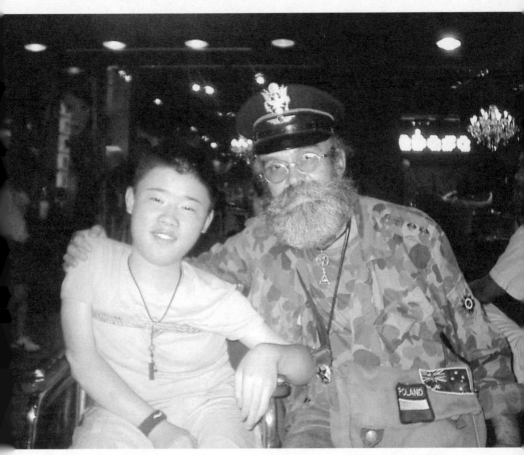

An Australian man asks for a photo with Huang Ge on the street in Guangzhou.

following 20-odd days. At the gloomiest of moments, the appearance of genuine kindness is immeasurably precious and unforgettable. Such kindness was also seen from other people. On the Huangs' way to Zhongshan City, a driver chased them for a long distance just to give them RMB 200.

The loss of their pedicab didn't ruin the Huangs' journey; instead, it exposed them to more love from their fellow citizens, which reinforced their determination to continue the Thanksgiving Journey. The world is made up of people both with soft hearts and those with hardened hearts. Based on their experiences, the Huangs believe the former far outnumber the latter.

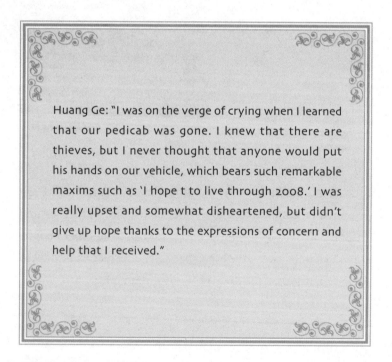

Huang Ge: "I was on the verge of crying when I learned that our pedicab was gone. I knew that there are thieves, but I never thought that anyone would put his hands on our vehicle, which bears such remarkable maxims such as 'I hope t to live through 2008.' I was really upset and somewhat disheartened, but didn't give up hope thanks to the expressions of concern and help that I received."

Risks and Dangers

The Huangs had a couple of brushes with death during their second Thanksgiving Journey.

One instance happened at the border region between Hunan and Guangdong provinces. In September, in pouring rain, the father and son plowed along a highway that spiraled up the mountain. As they went further into the mountain, there was less and less traffic on the road, and the gravel and rocks showered down from nearby slopes at the rumbling sounds of the engine. The road was slippery, and the abysm loomed on one side of the road. The father found it difficult to navigate the drive by himself, and said: "Son, the drive is getting more risky. I would like you to watch the right side, and guide me to stay away from the cliff, so that I can concentrate on dodging falling stones so that they don't fall on our vehicle." In this way the pair moved gingerly down the road, shifting between the brake and the accelerator. Whenever the crashing sounds made by falling rocks grew denser, the father had to slow down to reduce the engine's noise. It took them three hours to complete a 30 to 40 kilometer section of road.

Another adventure happened on another rainy day in No-

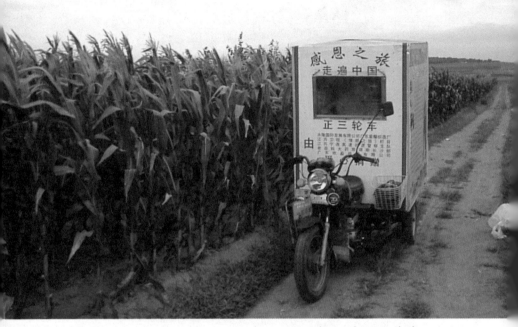

During their Thanksgiving Journey, the Huangs often rode on such dirt paths across crop fields.

vember on their way back to Hunan. The rain had lasted for several days. And due to a road repairing project, half of the lanes on the state highway between Yizhang and Chenzhou were closed. When the Huangs were halfway down a slope, a fully-loaded heavy truck came uphill towards them at full power from the opposite direction. Huang Xiaoyong immediately stopped his pedicab to give way to the jumbo truck. But the truck, in an attempt to stay away from the newly repaired lanes, kept pressing toward the Huangs. The pedicab was forced to move sideways until it was beyond the shoulder of the road, next to which was a gorge of 30 meters deep and

100 meters long. The pedicab inched toward the rim of the channel. In a panic Huang Xiaoyong jumped off his seat, planted his feet firmly into the muddy ground, and tried desperately to pull the vehicle back. But the sliding continued. When the rear tire was barely 50 cm from the cliff, he was sure he and his son were about to die. At this critical moment, amazingly, the movement of the vehicle was reversed. Not yet recovered from fright, Huang Xiaoyong spotted a few people running away from him and boarding a silver van, which soon disappeared in the rain. He then realized that these passengers had helped him haul the pedicab back onto the road. But he didn't see the van's license plate, and was therefore unable to find the names of his rescuers.

The Huangs feel fear when looking back at these hazardous

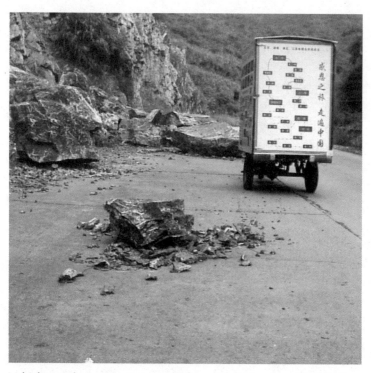

Vehicles on the mountain road at the border of Hunan and Guangdong provinces face great risks of having rocks pelt down on them from nearby cliffs.

moments in their journey, but at the same time, they feel a sense of triumph. They had foreseen the difficulties and dangers before setting off, but hadn't hesitated. They live by the rule of never submitting to adversity, which explains their struggle with illness and race with death over a period of so many years.

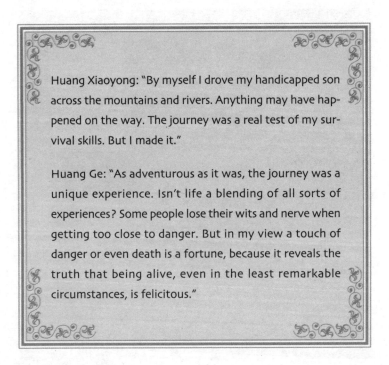

Huang Xiaoyong: "By myself I drove my handicapped son across the mountains and rivers. Anything may have happened on the way. The journey was a real test of my survival skills. But I made it."

Huang Ge: "As adventurous as it was, the journey was a unique experience. Isn't life a blending of all sorts of experiences? Some people lose their wits and nerve when getting too close to danger. But in my view a touch of danger or even death is a fortune, because it reveals the truth that being alive, even in the least remarkable circumstances, is felicitous."

The Third Thanksgiving Journey

During their previous two journeys, the Huangs had been the beneficiaries of much care and help from people. They were therefore inspired to pass on such kindnesses and encouragement to others in need. With this desire in mind, they planned their third journey.

Time: June 10 to August 11, 2006

Distance: 5,000 kilometers

Route: Changsha-Nanchang-Shangrao-Yiwu-Ningbo-Shaoxing-Hangzhou-Suzhou-Nantong-Yancheng-Lianyungang-Linyi-Zibo-Weifang-Yantai-Dalian-Anshan-Liaoyang-Shenyang-Tieling-Siping-Changchun-Harbin

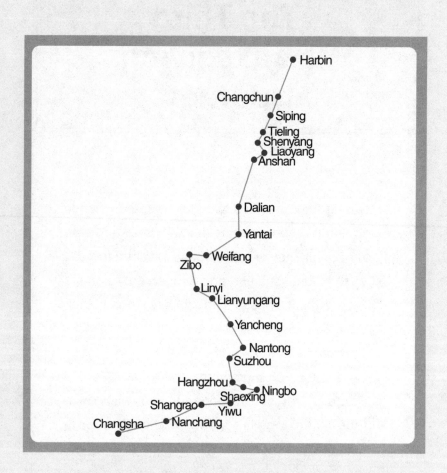

Meeting the Blind Girl Xinyue

In May 2005, much of the media across China reported the story of 8-year-old Xinyue of Changchun, Jilin Province. The girl had lost her eyesight and much of her mobility due to a deadly brain tumor. On learning of her desire to attend the flag-raising ceremony in Tian'anmen Square, more than 2000 people

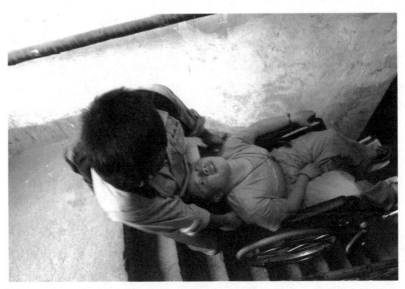

The father carries Huang Ge and his wheelchair up to a studio on the 8th floor to record a song for Xinyue.

in the city collaborated to simulate a trip to Beijing (as the girl was too weak to take a real trip) by recreating various sound effects that would normally have been heard on the train, bus and street on the way from Changchun to Beijing. When the national anthem was sung, and Xinyue was told she was in the square, she mirthfully made a salute with all her strength. The scenario was aired on TV to people around China, including the Huangs, bringing tears to every face. Huang Ge couldn't wait to see the girl on his next journey.

Huang Ge made by hand a flag of the Young Pioneers, a national schoolchildren's organization, and planned to collect signatures for the girl in every city he would visit on the way.

On learning of Huang Ge's desire to send the song *Forever* to Xinyue, a postgraduate student of the Central Conservatory of Music offered to help with the recording. The studio was on the eighth floor of a building without an elevator. Huang Ge in his wheelchair, with a combined weight of more than 74 kilograms, could not get there except by being carried by his father. The father stopped to have a break after climbing each floor, and took more than 40 minutes to reach the top.

During the singing Huang Ge choked at the lines "At the end of heaven or the other side of the ocean, my heart will always be with you; whenever it is or wherever I am, I pray for your health and happiness." This is exactly what Huang Ge wanted to tell not only Xinyue, but also everyone who cared about him. The boy was so focused on the singing that he was exhausted by the third taping of the recording, and had to stop. But the staff members praised him for his moving performance.

While his father did the packing for their third journey, Huang Ge laboriously typed his article "Let Love Ripple over China" on a computer.

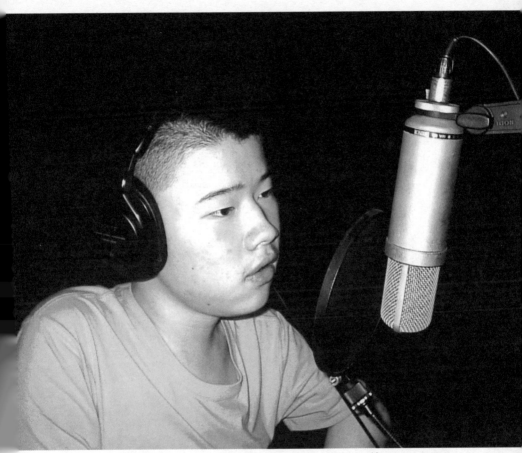

Huang Ge at the recording of his song *Forever*.

Huang Ge: "Doctors predict my life span to be 18 years. Eighteen years are ephemeral in human history, but the love that society and people have extended to me is infinite. It warms my heart, and has assured me that humanity prevails in this world. I want to relay this love to everyone seeking warmth, care, love and help."

Huang Xiaoyong: "I told my son that we could do something for Xinyue. We thought about how for a time, and then reached a consensus that it would be more meaningful to make a gift for her rather than to buy her one. At my suggestion my son made a Young Pioneers flag, and got the idea of collecting signatures for Xinyue along the way. By doing this we want to send her the message that most people in this world have a kind heart. We all love her and support her, and hope she can be strong in the coming days of her life."

Wavering Between Going on and Giving up

The Huangs started their third journey on an early summer day. Huang Ge asked his father to pin his article entitled "Let Love Ripple over China" on the cabin attached to the motorcycle.

The summer in southern China is wet and sultry. The sheet-iron cabin absorbed all the heat of the scorching sun, transforming the inside space into the equivalent of a sauna room. Huang Ge bounced in his wheelchair from the sudden impacts of the drive, sweating and panting. He had to ask his father to stop after driving one or two hours, so that he could get out to have some fresh air and stretch his limbs. To broaden the boy's field of vision, the father dismantled the windshield and the awning above his seat, exposing himself to slashing rain on bad-weather days and scorching sun on good-weather days.

Nobody knew of the father's pains and toils better than the son. To alleviate the burden on his father, Huang Ge tried to remain awake during the drive, so that he could manage to stay in the center of the cabin, and therefore keep the vehicle from lurching. When he saw a dent or bump on the road ahead, he would make a judgment about which direction the vehicle would tilt, and then prepare to throw himself in the opposite direction at the jolt. Being barely able to control his muscles, the boy however failed in many of the attempts, and had to try again at the next jolt.

The father, now 46, was overstraining himself. He drove during the day, and fluttered a fan at night to keep mosquitoes away from the boy. To make things worse, his motorcycle malfunctioned from time to time owing to the long drive and hot weather. And for much of the time, the search for donors didn't go smoothly. For too often the addresses were inaccurate, and the telephone numbers had changed, leaving the Huangs few clues as to the whereabouts of their benefactors.

When they reached Hangzhou, Huang Xiaoyong felt he had reached the physical and psychological limits of his strength. In poor health, with a tatty motorcycle and no money in his pocket, he saw no reason to go on with the trip, and considered selling the vehicle and returning home. Huang Ge was confronted with a difficult choice. On the one hand he could well understand how his father felt. On the other hand, he, months away from his 18th birthday, the predicted end-point of his life, was more conscious of the threat of death, but still held fast to

To keep smiling, remain optimistic and never give up, are Huang Ge's life principles.

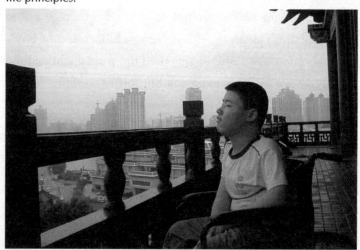

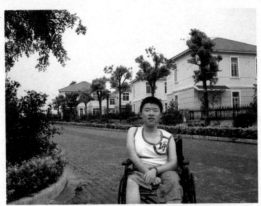

Huang Ge in the Jiangxiang New Village in the prosperous suburbs of Changzhou City, Jiangsu Province.

a glitter of hope that a miracle might happen during the trip. He secretly hoped: "Maybe someday, someplace along the way I may find a cure for my disease…"

Huang Ge decided to have a man-to-man talk with his father. He quoted a sentence he had learnt from TV: Not every effort yields positive results, but giving up leads to sure failure. Huang Xiaoyong had not known that his son could be so sophisticated, and wept for the first time in front of the boy. They resumed the trip northward, collecting signatures for Xinyue on the way.

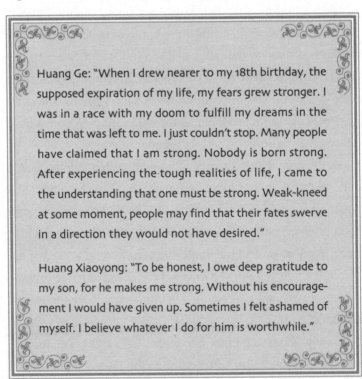

Huang Ge: "When I drew nearer to my 18th birthday, the supposed expiration of my life, my fears grew stronger. I was in a race with my doom to fulfill my dreams in the time that was left to me. I just couldn't stop. Many people have claimed that I am strong. Nobody is born strong. After experiencing the tough realities of life, I came to the understanding that one must be strong. Weak-kneed at some moment, people may find that their fates swerve in a direction they would not have desired."

Huang Xiaoyong: "To be honest, I owe deep gratitude to my son, for he makes me strong. Without his encouragement I would have given up. Sometimes I felt ashamed of myself. I believe whatever I do for him is worthwhile."

A Five-yuan Donation with Two-yuan Change

"We experienced both the bad and good during our trips," said Huang Ge. "At first I didn't understand why the drivers passing by on the state highways honked their horns twice. Later my father told me that their honking represented their cheers for us." A caring look, a smile or a bottle of water, every bit of kindness offered to the father and son touched their hearts.

The trips were completely funded by donations. The Huangs were out of money once again when they were in Yueyang. The local media helped them with a fundraising event in a busy district, which attracted a large number of people.

In the crowd stood a ragged woman with a tanned face, a carrying pole in one hand and a little girl in the other. She watched for half an hour before walking away in silence, but soon returned with a timid expression. "This five yuan is all I have. I just want to give you three yuan, could you give me change of two yuan?" She dropped the crumpled note into the donation box, and took out two one-yuan notes with a quivering hand.

Huang Xiaoyong burst into tears at the sight. The mother and daughter were no better off than the Huangs, but looked

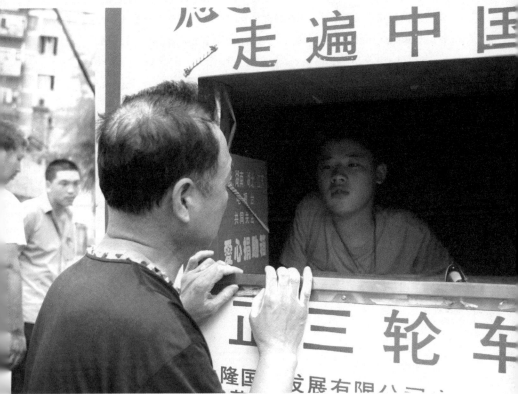

People would stop to convey their greetings to Huang Ge as soon as they saw him.

mirthful on doing their best to help others. He caught up with them, and tucked his last ten yuan into the little girl's pocket.

The woman is in fact one of the many people who spared a sum for the Huangs from their meager incomes. Another example is Mr. Yuan Xiaowei in Suzhou. On seeing him, the Huangs were taken aback that Mr. Yuan, in his 60s, took odd jobs after retirement to support himself and his chronically ill mother who was in the 90s. Even in such circumstances, Yuan managed to save money for poor college students.

It is easier for the rich to offer financial help to others. Compared with what they have their giving is merely a drop in the ocean. That's why some magnates see charity as a handy method to polish their public images. But it is always real affection and mercy that motivate the poor to share their few possessions with others. Such help is the best embodiment of human kindness.

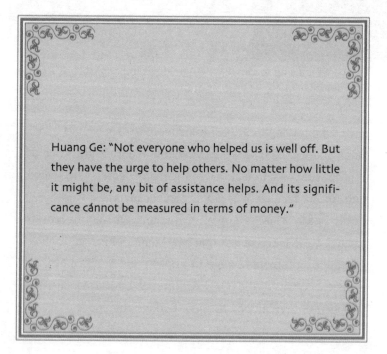

Huang Ge: "Not everyone who helped us is well off. But they have the urge to help others. No matter how little it might be, any bit of assistance helps. And its significance cánnot be measured in terms of money."

Signatures and Blessings of the Dalian People

In early July 2006, the Huangs reached Dalian, but didn't find the two donors in the city, who had changed their telephone numbers.

Then the father and son worked to collect signatures from the locals for the blind girl Xinyue. They first contacted the local media, describing their plan to collect signatures in the

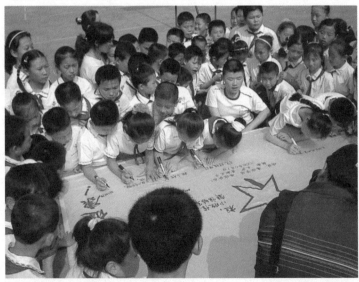

Children write down their blessings for Xinyue on a Young Pioneer Flag.

city's Children's Center. They didn't go to the center themselves because of a previous failed experience. In their hometown Changsha, they had gone to Hunan University with the same request, but were rejected by skeptical cadres. They since learnt to seek the media's assistance for similar events.

In the Dalian Children's Center, Huang Ge told the story of Xinyue to its teachers and students. At the end of his speech, they jostled forward to leave their names on the flag, together with their blessings for the father and son. The ebullient scene reminded the Huangs of another case in a Hangzhou primary school. It had been noon. The schoolmaster had summoned more than 100 students in the playground as student representatives. They moved in a queue toward the Young Pioneer flag unfurled on a table tennis table, and solemnly signed their names. Such scenes were repeated during the Huangs' third Thanksgiving Journey.

If love is a flame, it should be bundled into a torch, and relayed to as many people as possible, kindling virtues in every heart. Love is at the core of humanity, which serves as the cornerstone of civilization.

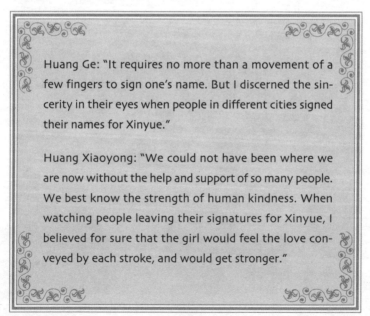

Huang Ge: "It requires no more than a movement of a few fingers to sign one's name. But I discerned the sincerity in their eyes when people in different cities signed their names for Xinyue."

Huang Xiaoyong: "We could not have been where we are now without the help and support of so many people. We best know the strength of human kindness. When watching people leaving their signatures for Xinyue, I believed for sure that the girl would feel the love conveyed by each stroke, and would get stronger."

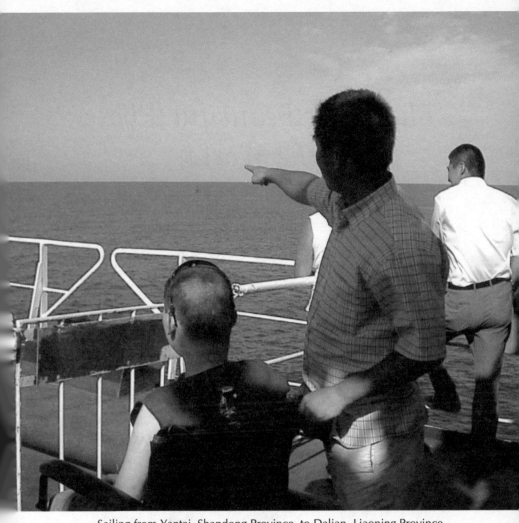

Sailing from Yantai, Shandong Province, to Dalian, Liaoning Province.

The Most Beautiful Eyes in the World

On the next stop, Shenyang, the Huangs got the news that Xinyue was to leave for Beijing in a few days for medical treatment. They rushed to Changchun as fast as they could to see the girl before her departure.

Having so much to say before meeting Xinyue, Huang Ge couldn't remember anything when he eventually came to her bed. The girl, who had recently undergone an operation couldn't

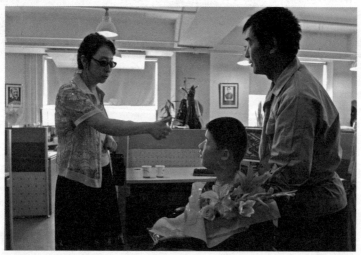

A donor in Changchun, Jilin Province, gives a thumbs-up to Huang Ge during their meeting.

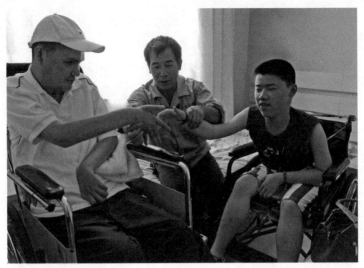

The Huangs cheer on a man who has been paralyzed by a traffic accident.

speak clearly or make any expression properly due to the paralysis on the left side of her face. But she tried to greet the Huangs with a smile. Huang Ge held her hands, and shed tears.

The Huangs placed into the girl's arms the Young Pioneer flag with the signatures, a CD of the song *Forever* sung by Huang Ge himself, and various gifts from people they had met

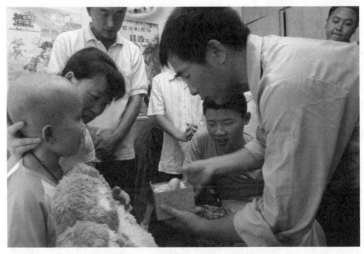

The Huangs pass to Xinyue the gifts people have entrusted to them during their trip.

along the way. The blind girl ran her hands across these presents, and put on a smile as well as she could.

Huang Ge wrote about his meeting with the girl on his blog:

"At the first sight of Xinyue I knew her condition was worse than I had expected. But she had the most beautiful eyes in the world, so clear and so honest. I was bitterful that God must

Huang Ge with Xinyue, the girl who has lost her eyesight to a brain tumor.

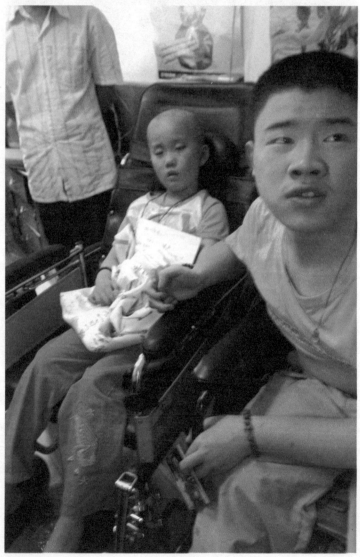

have lost His sight if he could wield such a blow to a girl like Xinyue. I hoped she could create a miracle as I had. I was told by doctors that my life would be no longer than 18 years, but I am still alive now. The doctors have also concluded that Xinyue is very ill. But if they could make one mistake, they might make another one. I do wish Xinyue a happy and long life."

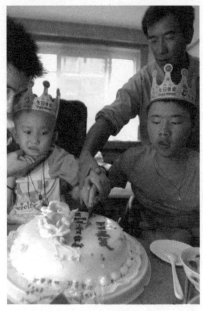

Huang Ge and Xinyue cut a cake with the assistance of others.

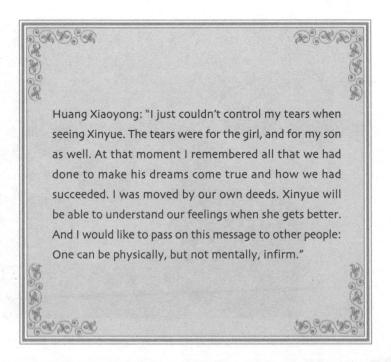

Huang Xiaoyong: "I just couldn't control my tears when seeing Xinyue. The tears were for the girl, and for my son as well. At that moment I remembered all that we had done to make his dreams come true and how we had succeeded. I was moved by our own deeds. Xinyue will be able to understand our feelings when she gets better. And I would like to pass on this message to other people: One can be physically, but not mentally, infirm."

Reaching the Finish Line

On August 13, 2006, the Huangs arrived in Harbin, the last stop on their third Thanksgiving Journey.

August is the best season in the northeastern Chinese city. And the Huangs met most of their donors there. The third Thanksgiving Journey had a perfect ending. To give them more

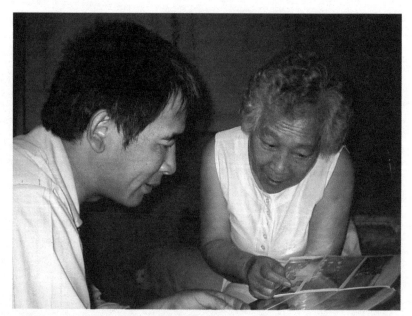

Showing photos to a donor's mother.

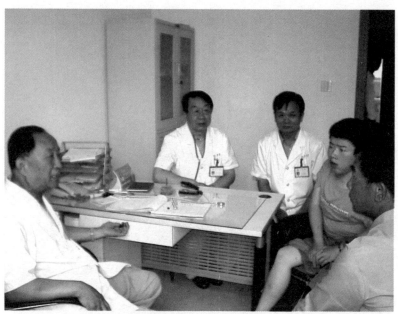

Doctors from a hospital in Harbin, Heilongjiang Province, determine a group diagnosis for Huang Ge.

pleasure, the local pharmaceutical company Heibao offered them a tour to their bear farm, the largest in the world with a bear population of 1,500, in the neighboring Mudanjiang City. The father and son frolicked with the bear cubs on the lawn, and fed them.

The Huangs returned to Changsha by air. Their motorcycle had come to the verge of collapse after the long trip. But the owner of a local motorcycle shop still offered to buy it at RMB 1,000, apparently for philanthropic purposes.

When the plane landed at the Huanghua Airport in Changsha, the Huangs felt as if they were back to reality after a dream. Over the previous three years they had toured around more than 80 cities in China, looking for their donors to convey their thanks

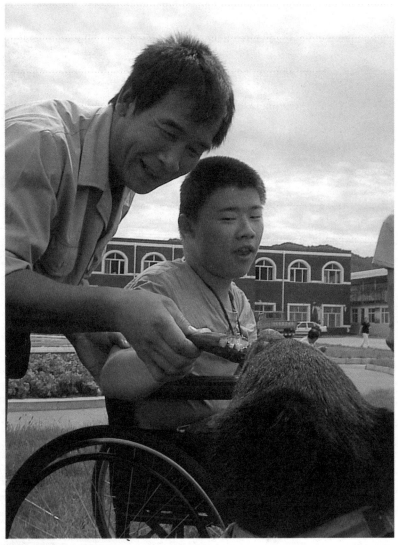

Playing with a baby bear at a bear farm.

personally. The odyssey would have been an ordeal for people of sound body, not to mention a boy with a severe disability and his impecunious father. For the Huangs the bitterness and hardships they endured on the way are merely episodes that give greater prominence to the generous love people extended to them and the confidence and self-fulfillment they achieved as a result of the experience.

Huang Ge: "There is a Chinese saying: traveling brings one broader knowledge than reading. I think this is true. After seeing so many places with my father, I have grown more mature than others of my age, as I have experienced more in life. I have been deprived of many things since childhood: mother's love, the companionship of classmates and free actions. But meanwhile I have been blessed with things that some people may never have in their lives."

Huang Xiaoyong: "The plane arrived in Changsha a few hours after taking off in Harbin. But it had taken us several months to cover the distance on our vehicle. I had a strange feeling when the plane touched the ground, and I didn't know whether it was happiness or bitterness. The world is small, as I can go around China on a bike. To one of strong will, nothing is impossible. Whatever you do, you can never make it if you only focus on the difficulties that may occur.

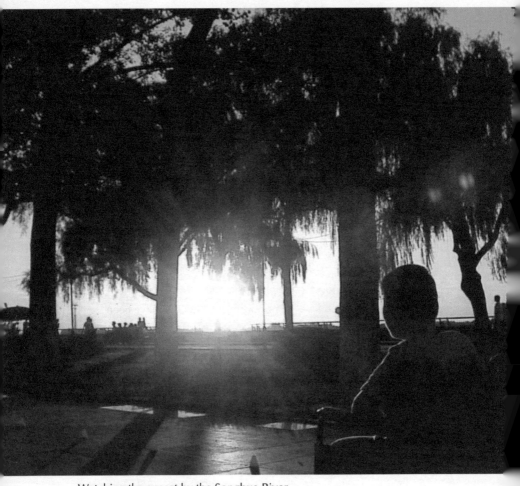

Watching the sunset by the Songhua River.

IV. 18th Birthday

Huang Ge mocked death, which threatened to take him before the age of 18. He was cheerfully and confidently approaching the predicted age of doom. Though he is confined to his wheelchair (where he has to be fastened by a belt in order to keep himself upright) and bed, he keeps his mind wide open, and strives for his dreams.

Three Celebrations for the 18th Birthday

October 30, 2006, was Huang Ge's 18th birthday, a date doctors predicted he might never reach.

The father and son began to plan for a grand celebration for the date one month in advance, which they hoped would be attended by all their friends, neighbors and relatives. Then came the call from the CCTV talk show Telling the Truth, inviting them to Beijing.

On October 27, the Huangs showed up in the production room of the program in Beijing. The staff members had arranged a birthday party for the boy ahead of his actual birthday. When the music was played, the host brought to Huang Ge a cake with the pattern of a cerulean ocean, golden sailboat and splendid flowers, the most beautiful cake he had ever seen. His father and the host held his hand to cut the cake. To give him a bigger surprise, the staff dialed the number of Yi Zhongtian (a professor of history whose lectures on TV drew throngs of fans across China), who was an idol of Huang Ge. On hearing Prof. Yi say that he considered Huang Ge to be his teacher, the boy beamed with delight and pride.

On October 30, the Huangs were still in Beijing. On recalling their journey to Tian'anmen Square on their pedicab three years earlier, they decided to re-visit the site on this special day. And the experience was as sweet as the previous one had been. In the evening a local resident called, offering them a treat for the boy's birthday. They had a hearty meal in a restaurant serving authentic Hunan cuisine. The food was so good that Huang Ge had more than his stomach could handle. A severe stomachache struck around 3 am the next morning, and his father had to rush him to a hospital emergency room.

Uttering a wish at his 18th birthday party.

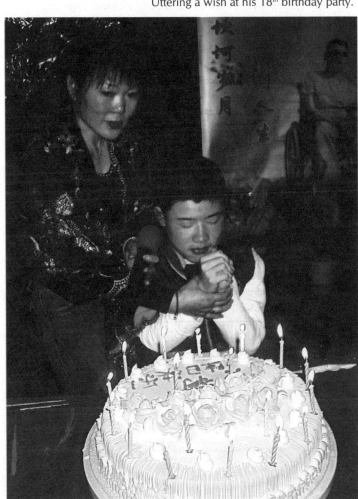

The episode of Telling the Truth about the Huangs' story was aired on December 10, when the Huangs hosted another party at home in Changsha to celebrate the fact that Huang Ge had reached his 18th year.

For Huang Ge, no dainty morsels tasted better than the birthday cake of the day, as it was the trophy of his triumph in the battle against death. Knowing one's possible date with doom is devastating for every mortal. Huang Ge, instead of succumbing to his fate, exerts himself to bring the utmost value and meaning to every minute of his life. He isn't sure if there is any medicine in the world that can cure his disease, but he is convinced that one's willpower has even better remedial effects than medicine, as it is the only power that can hold back the steps of death.

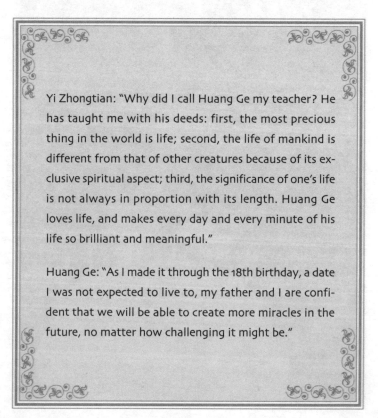

Yi Zhongtian: "Why did I call Huang Ge my teacher? He has taught me with his deeds: first, the most precious thing in the world is life; second, the life of mankind is different from that of other creatures because of its exclusive spiritual aspect; third, the significance of one's life is not always in proportion with its length. Huang Ge loves life, and makes every day and every minute of his life so brilliant and meaningful."

Huang Ge: "As I made it through the 18th birthday, a date I was not expected to live to, my father and I are confident that we will be able to create more miracles in the future, no matter how challenging it might be."

A "Sunny Boy" That Moves China

On February 26, 2007, Huang Ge was elected one of the ten "Figures That Have Moved China" of the year 2006.

At the awards ceremony, Huang Xiaoyong rejected the offer of help by staff members, and by himself carried Huang Ge in his wheelchair up the stairs to the stage. Every step was difficult, but was no more difficult than the days he had lived through in previous years. No one could share the bitterness he

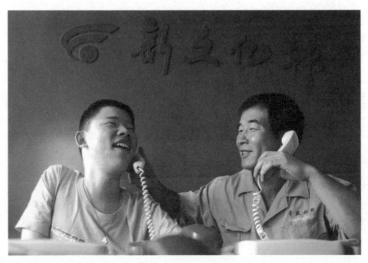

A kind utterance gives the Huangs enormous joy and comfort.

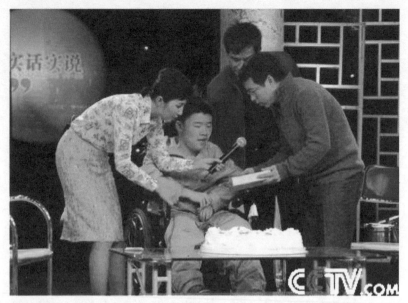

Huang Ge receives a gift on the site of the production of the CCTV talk show Telling the Truth.

experienced in the past, nor the joy he felt at that moment. He preferred to keep his emotions to himself. When the Huangs stood on the stage, thunderous applause broke out. The father held the son's hands to wave to the audience, and tears poured down their faces.

The emcee had the following conversation with the pair:

Emcee: "In the past you were moved by others, and meanwhile moved people."

Huang Ge: "Yes. I think the fact that we have won the honor of "Moving China" is the best repayment for those who have helped us. It's their encouragement and support that have enabled us to be where we are now. So we owe much gratitude to them."

Emcee: "How do you feel different before and after saying thanks to them?"

Huang Ge: "I would be ashamed if I didn't know the names, gender or ages of our helpers; when I went to thank them personally, I let them know that I take their kindness to heart."

Emcee: "What prompted you to change from one being aided

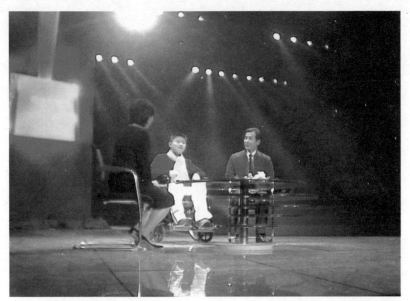
Taking questions from the emcee at the awards ceremony for Moving China 2006.

to one aiding others?"

Huang Ge: "I know there are many people in the world who are more unfortunate than I am. The care and support I have received from the public have changed my life, so I got the urge to help others and to disseminate this message: anyone in need can get help in this society, and everyone who has received help from others should not forget such kindness…"

During their Thanksgiving Journey, the Huangs never thought they would someday come to the "Moving China" awards stage. As they carried on city by city on the pedicab to acknowledge the help of people, they started a relay of love and compassion.

Cross-country Lecture Tour

After the story of the Huangs was told across China, people drew courage from them in coping with the unpleasant and unfortunate aspects of life. From February to June 2007, the father and son were invited to a dozen speeches, sharing with huge crowds their experiences and thoughts and preaching passion and hope in life.

On March 13, Huang Ge made the following remarks to an

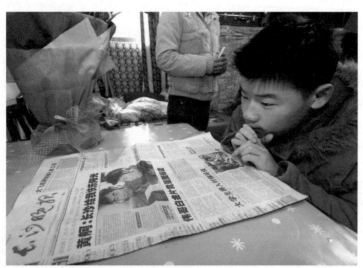

Huang Ge reads a report about his father and him in the newspaper.

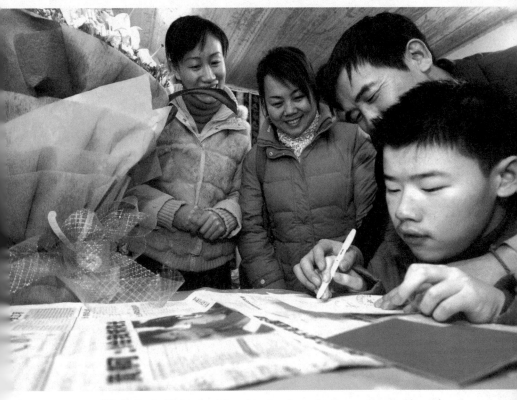

The father holds his son's hand to sign for a charity program in Changsha, Hunan Province.

audience of 800 of his age group at a gathering themed "How Will We Grow up Today?" at the Luwan Educational, Cultural and Sports Center in Shanghai:

"To be honest, I am jealous of you, my brothers and sisters. You may groan that there are many troubles in life. But in the eyes of someone like me, even something as simple as attending a class is so admirable and desperately impossible. So please be happy with what you have and what you are undergoing now, as they are all the gifts of life. I didn't know this until losing too much in my life. Why don't you appreciate their value while you have them? So you don't have to have regrets in later years."

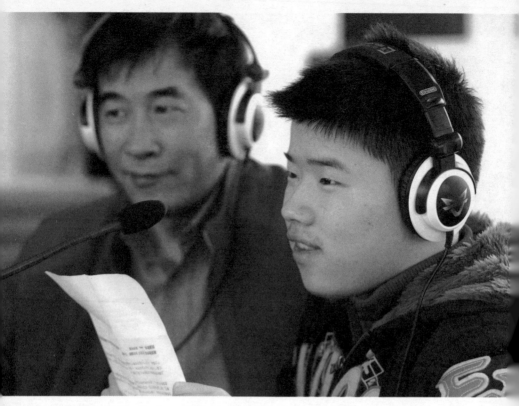

The Huangs talk about their views on life on a program produced by Hunan Radio.

"We Are Moved by the Nation"

A student: "Huang Ge, on winning the "Moving China" award, who do you think actually moved the nation, you or your father?"

Huang Ge: "We didn't move the nation; instead, we are moved by the nation. It was the generous help provided to us by so many kind people that inspired and enabled us to make the Thanksgiving Journey, and instilled optimism in me. If you insist on having me make a choice between my father and me, it is my father. With my disability, I could have done nothing without assistance. My father, after losing everything he had, keeps alive his hopes, and has remained by my side. Though the "Moving China" award was granted to me, it is my father who truly deserves it."

"The Breadth of Life Is Unlimited"

A student: "I have a question for Huang Ge. What was your achievement during the Thanksgiving Journey?"

Huang Ge: "The concern the public showed for me is my largest gain from the trip. To be more realistic, the trip itself is of the greatest benefit to me. My life may be cut short at 20 or younger, but I could have lived a richer life than many who live longer, as I have seen so many people and gone through so many happenings. The length of life is limited, but the breadth of live is unlimited."

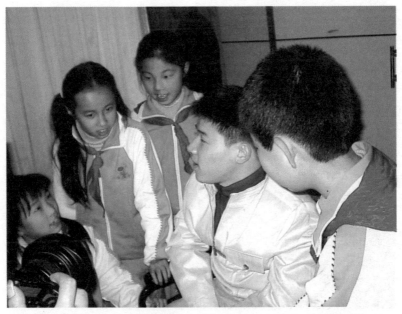

Huang Ge exchanges words with children of his age.

"I Will Always Be Happy in the Coming Years"

A student: "Do you still feel happy after experiencing so many adversities?"

Huang Ge: "I am happy, now and forever. My happiness is the best compensation for my father and for all people who have helped me. Every day and in every circumstance I will keep smiles on my face."

"I'll Make Every Day of My Life a Miracle"

A student: "I have a question for Huang Ge. What's your plan for the future?"

Huang Ge: Nothing in particular. I have always believed that what happens in the future is unpredictable, but what we do can effect change. I am going to make every day of my life a miracle, and by doing so ensure that everything that my fa-

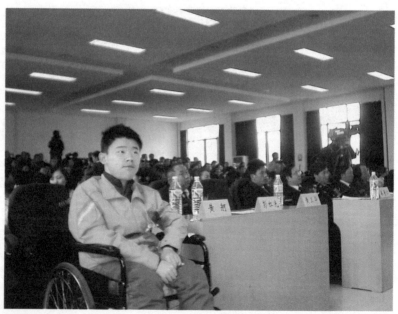

The Huangs at a gathering themed Learning from Lei Feng.

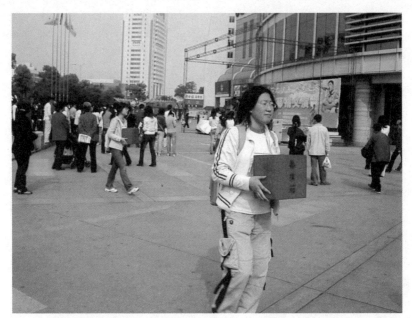

Inspired by Huang Ge, students of Hunan University collect donations for a charity program Moral Bank.

ther has done for me isn't a waste of time, and that I am as strong as possible."

...

Many people may blame others or fate when they find themselves in adverse situations, and many lose heart when encountering setbacks. In front of the Huangs they will find how trivial their troubles are and how lucky they have been. There is no reason for them not to take life as it is, cheerfully and gratefully.

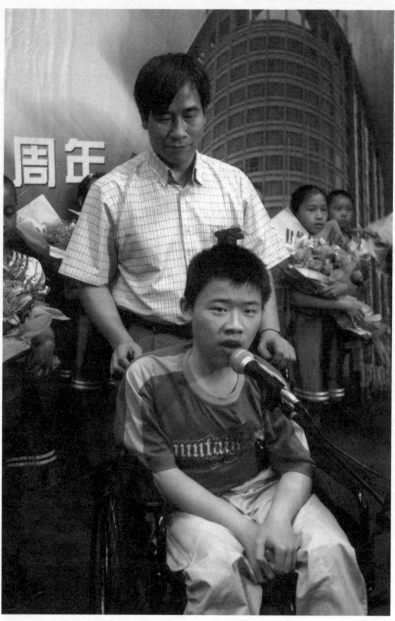

The Huangs are ardent about various social welfare activities.

"He Is a Considerate Boy"

The erosion of Huang Ge's health caused by his disease is more and more evident. His spine now twists like an "S," making it impossible for him to lie on his back. During sleep he has to stay on one side for hours, then ask his father to turn him over onto the other side. His body is very sore after remaining in one position for too long.

An uninterrupted sleep therefore seems an unreachable luxury for the father. The father and son share a bed. At three or four every morning, the boy has to awaken his father to turn him over. No matter how reluctant he may be to open his eyes, the father has to answer his son's call, as the boy needs him. "To be honest, I felt I'd had enough of it at some point."

Giving the boy a shower is also a great headache, particularly in winter, when their shabby home is chilly. The father has to wear rain boots before undressing the boy and taking him to the bathroom. Being inert for too long, the boy often has bedsores. His father gives him an overall check after each shower, and dabs medicine on the ulcerous spots. The whole process takes more than one hour. And at the end of it both father and son are shivering because of the cold.

Huang Ge has been a sweet boy since childhood. When he lived with his grandparents in the early years, he was always the one who kept laughter in the room. If he saw that the adults were busy, he never bothered them even when he was hungry. Instead, he would wait in silence. After he lost his mobility to the disease, his considerate trait became even more conspicuous. For instance, to alleviate the burden on his father, he drank as little water as possible to reduce his visits to the bathroom. When the dog-tired father fell asleep after toiling during the day, Huang Ge would turn the TV volume as low as possible, and wouldn't utter a word until his bladder was ready to burst.

For years the Huangs lived by the same schedule everyday: watch TV until midnight, and then sleep to noon of the following day. By doing so they could skip the breakfast meal. In order to save some money to buy more and better food for his son, the father eventually gave up his supper, surviving on one

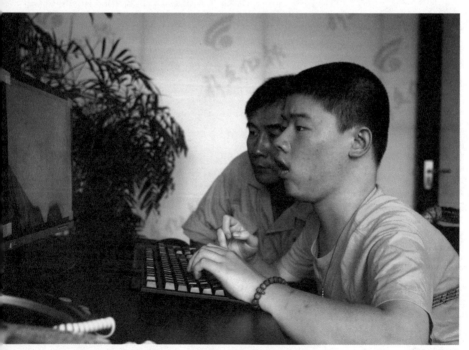

Father and son always together doing everything.

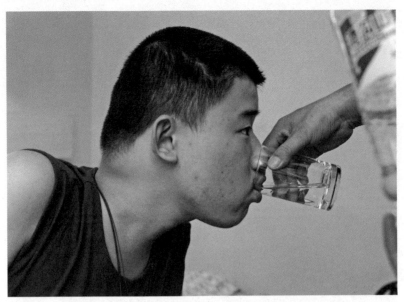

Even giving the boy a drink demands utmost care and great skill.

meal daily. But to give his home-bound son some entertainment, he scratched together the sum needed to purchase a TV, their only valuable possession, and managed to refurbish the interior of their rental home. "My son was encaged in these rooms for months and years. I felt obliged to do all I could to make his life more comfortable."

It is not difficult to imagine how a man feels when he has to give up his career in his prime years and play nanny to his sick son every minute of the day. But after seeing the concerns and attachment the boy showed for him when enduring a consumptive disease, all his grievances were dissipated. Depending on each other year after year, the Huangs felt the bond between them grow stronger and stronger.

Giving the boy a wash.

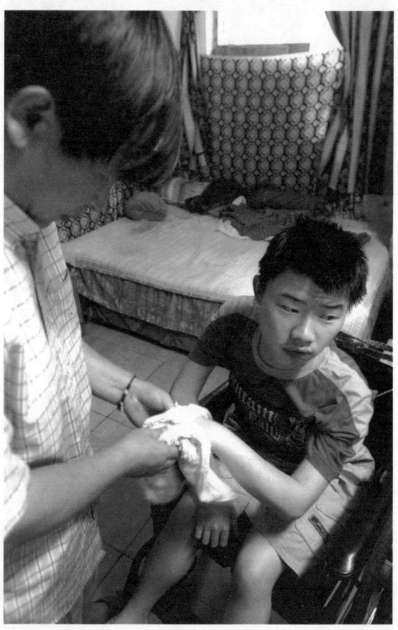

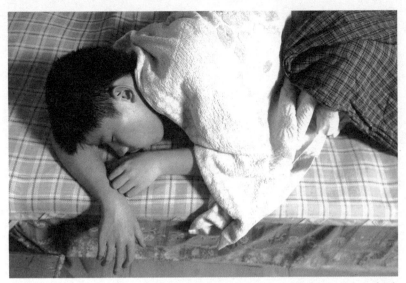

Only in this position can Huang Ge feel less pain in bed.

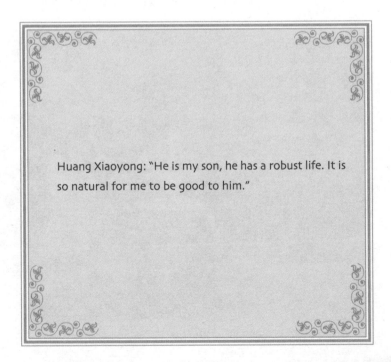

Huang Xiaoyong: "He is my son, he has a robust life. It is so natural for me to be good to him."

Simple Fun

For most of the time at home Huang Ge sits in his wheelchair in their one-story humble house watching TV, which offers him a window on the outside world. He likes investigative news programs the most, and knows the first run and re-run times for each. Sometimes the father and son enjoy a movie on

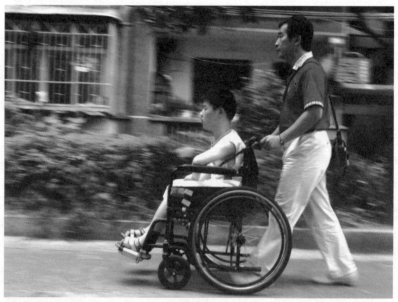

The father pushes his son to a lecture site.

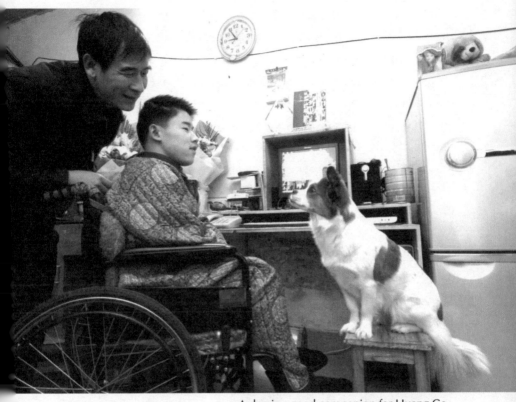

A dog is a good companion for Huang Ge.

VCD. To create a home theater effect, the father installed two sound boxes on the back wall opposite the TV. From time to time they have a small concert on their crackly karaoke machine.

On his 18th birthday, a businessman sent Huang Ge a computer. Despite the difficulty in commanding his fingers, the boy soon taught himself how to use it and log onto the Internet. His vision has since been broadened. The Internet gives him access to a bigger world. He later created a blog to post his articles on his deeds and thoughts. Each entry takes several hours. He has made friends on the net, and chats with them to exchange encouraging words. Computer games are also a good means of killing time. His favorite game is car racing. Seeing his car dash down the course across obstacles, he has the illusion that he is running with it.

Since recording the song *Forever*, Huang Ge has aspired to someday be a musician. And he feels hopeful about reaching this goal with the help of his computer and the Internet.

From time to time the Huangs review the photos they took during their Thanksgiving Journey, recalling their days on the

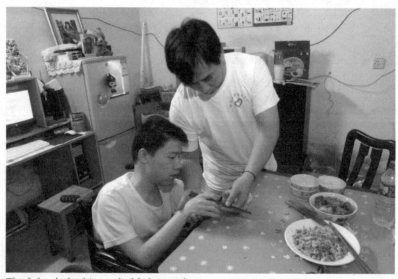

The father helps his son hold chopsticks.

trip. As more people have since helped them, they say that the journey has not yet come to an end.

Huang Ge plans to donate his corneas when death eventually snatches him. He is not afraid of death, but hopes it will come as late as possible so that he can still realize more dreams. Sometimes he wakes up suddenly in the night, and cannot fall asleep again. Then he prays for more time in this world, and promises to make the best use of every minute.

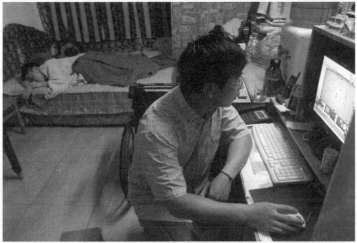

The father briefly relaxes when his son is sleeping.

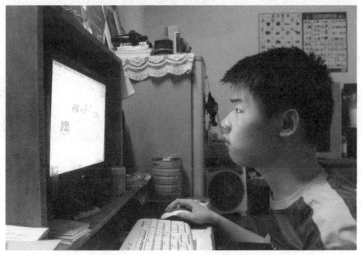

Huang Ge has taught himself to use the computer.

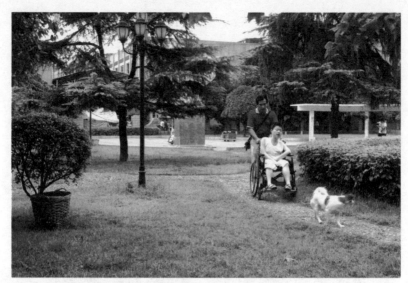

The father and son and their dog strolling in a park.

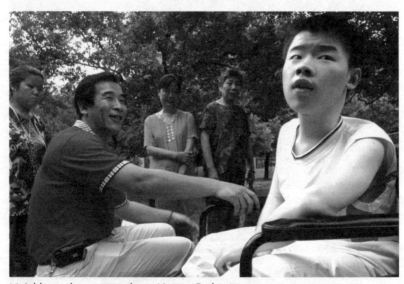

Neighbors always try to keep Huang Ge happy.

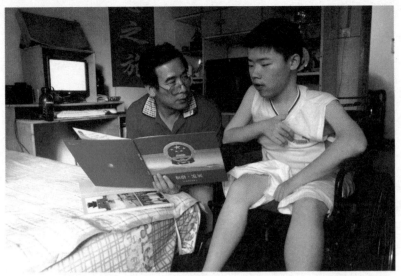

The Huangs keep volumes of photos from their Thanksgiving Journey.

Huang Ge: "Since I came into this world, I have had to accept life as it is, and make the best of it. Everyone will die, so there is no need to bother with the thought about when one is going to die. What is most important is to live a life without regrets. So at the end of it one can leave in peace and with a smile."

Huang Xiaoyong: "At this stage of his illness, I don't want to evade, or have my son evade, what's going to happen. My biggest desire is to make him happy every hour of every day. His happiness is the whole meaning of my life. In order to create a fruitful and delightful life for him, I have been planning and dreaming with him. We have several dreams at present, and will soon put them into action. I hope we will still have time."

Postscript

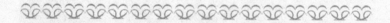

"Saying Thanks at the End of Life." When I wrote down these words, my eyes were blurred with tears, and I felt a charge go through my body.

Most people would judge that the blows of life have plunged the Huangs into a situation where the soil for hope is barren. But to their amazement, the father and son have cultivated a brilliant blossom on it with extraordinary adamancy and persistence, sending the message of hope to millions of hearts.

The explanation for the miracle may possibly be found in Huang Ge's words: "One must be grateful for life, grateful for the bare fact that one is living, and for every bit of care and help one receives." I believe this is the secret behind why the boy has been smiling throughout all the mishaps in his young life, and has preserved the strength to love others.

When reflecting on the past 13 years since Huang Ge was diagnosed with muscular dystrophy, it is clear that

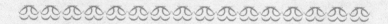

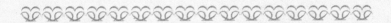

the Huangs display a peace of mind that can only be found in those who have survived a tempest.

For Huang Ge, each day marks a step closer to death, but he and his father are unperturbed, as if they have forgotten the imminent threat. Instead they are occupied with plans to do more meaningful things. Jeff Blatnick, a wrestler with cancer who won an Olympic gold medal, once said that though every one would lose the battle against death sooner or later, he would keep moving forward even when he was on the verge of death. This is exactly what Huang Ge has lived up to.

Everyone who knows any people as brave and tough as the Huangs prays for time to go at its slowest pace, so that Huang Ge may realize more of his dreams. He has vowed that he will never give up as long as his brain continues to function.

图书在版编目（CIP）数据

在生命的最后说"谢谢"：英文/方雯著． －北京：外文出版社，2008
ISBN 978-7-119-05490-2

Ⅰ．在… Ⅱ．方… Ⅲ．①英语-语言读物 ②长篇小说-中国-
当代 Ⅳ.H319.4：I

中国版本图书馆 CIP 数据核字(2008)第 108887 号

策　　　划：兰佩瑾
撰　　　文：方　雯
摄　　　影：明健飞　刘　军等
翻　　　译：孙　蕾　雨秋
英 文 审 稿：Solange Dilverberg　汪光强
印 刷 监 制：冯　浩
责 任 编 辑：兰佩瑾　文　芳

在生命的最后说"谢谢"

© 外文出版社
外文出版社出版
（中国北京百万庄大街24号）
邮政编码：100037
外文出版社网页：http://www.flp.com.cn
北京外文印刷厂印刷
中国国际图书贸易总公司发行
（中国北京车公庄西路35号）
北京邮政信箱第399号 邮政编码100044
2008 年(小 16 开)第 1 版
2008 年第 1 版第 1 次印刷
（英文）
ISBN 978-7-119-05490-2
06800（平）
10-E-3884P